Neuropsychiatry Case Studies

Josef Priller • Hugh Rickards
Editors

Neuropsychiatry Case Studies

Springer

Editors
Josef Priller
Department of Neuropsychiatry
Charité – Universitätsmedizin Berlin
Berlin
Germany

Hugh Rickards
Birmingham and Solihull MHFT
Birmingham University
Edgbaston, Birmingham
UK

ISBN 978-3-319-42188-9 ISBN 978-3-319-42190-2 (eBook)
DOI 10.1007/978-3-319-42190-2

Library of Congress Control Number: 2016960001

Printed on acid-free paper

This Springer imprint is published by Springer Nature
The registered company is Springer International Publishing AG
The registered company address is: Gewerbestrasse 11, 6330 Cham, Switzerland

Preface

In a narrow definition, neuropsychiatry deals with cognitive, emotional and behavioural problems of neurological disorders. We have asked eminent neuropsychiatrists from around the world to provide us with a case study that has taught them an important lesson or has influenced their clinical care. The result is a collection of cases that pay tribute to the diversity of neuropsychiatry.

The case observations are meant to inspire the reader. We hope that they stimulate curiosity and further exploration. The book contains excellent examples of neuropsychiatric assessment and treatment approaches. However, we do not provide a comprehensive overview of neuropsychiatry, nor does the book contain the latest scientific discoveries.

Neuropsychiatry has a long tradition in Europe. The discipline has now been established worldwide to provide the clinical skills that are required to link brain structure and function. The authors of this book come from three continents and ten different countries. They share an enthusiasm for neuropsychiatry, which we hope you will enjoy.

Berlin, Germany — Josef Priller
Edgbaston, Birmingham, UK — Hugh Rickards

Contents

Part I Dementias

1 **Unexplained Delirium, Atypical Dementia, and Prodromal DLB** ... 3
Ian McKeith

2 **Unable to Talk** ... 7
Fernando Lázaro Perlado

3 **A Mistaken Recurrent Depression** ... 13
Eike Jakob Spruth

4 **An Atypical Variant of a Common Neurodegenerative Disorder** ... 17
Adith Mohan, Teresa Lee, and Perminder Sachdev

5 **Posterior Cortical Atrophy (PCA)** ... 25
Tillmann Supprian

6 **Case Study: Little Red Riding Hood** ... 31
Marlies Baldee-Hordijk and Erik van Duijn

7 **Not All Unusual Behavior Is Psychotic** ... 37
Kevin Foy

8 **Puzzling Case: Is the Answer in the Genes?** ... 41
Emma Devenney and John Hodges

Part II Movement Disorders

9 **Hallucinations in Parkinson's Disease** ... 49
Roger A. Barker and Gemma Cummins

10 **Parkinsons and Parasomnias** ... 55
Hugh Selsick

11 **The Possible Talents of Tourette Syndrome** 61
Andrea E. Cavanna

12 **On the Nature of Separation Challenges and Attachment Solutions in Severe, Refractory Gilles de la Tourette Syndrome (GTS): Deep Brain Stimulation (DBS) Has Been Helpful, But What About Rikki and Luci and Now Riley?** 67
James F. Leckman

13 **Paroxysmal Disorders in Autism: Problems with Diagnosis and Management** 75
Kanu Achinivu

14 **Twitches and Fidgets Might Not Tell the Whole Story** 81
Mary May Robertson, Valsamma Eapen, and Renata Rizzo

15 **Apathy in Huntington's Disease: Medicating the Patient, Spouse, Both, or None?** 89
Harald Gelderblom

Part III Functional Disorders

16 **Diagnostic Layers** 95
Tiago Teodoro and Mark J. Edwards

17 **A Case of a Familial "Dopamine-Responsive" Movement Disorder** 99
J.M. Gelauff and M.A.J. de Koning-Tijssen

18 **Facial Spasm Can Look Like Facial Weakness in Patients with Functional Disorders** 103
Jon Stone

19 **Review of Notes Documenting Initial Treatment Is Crucial in the Assessment of Acquired Brain Injury** 109
Killian Welch

Part IV Epilepsy and Psychogenic Nonepileptic Seizures

20 **Novel Seizure Semiology After Epilepsy Surgery** 115
Martin Holtkamp

21 **The Syndrome of Transient Epileptic Amnesia** 121
Adam Zeman

22 **Autobiographical Amnesia in Association with Subtle Temporal Lobe Seizures** 127
Christopher R. Butler

23 **A Diagnostic Challenge of Troublesome Nocturnal Episodes** 131
Frank Besag

24 Past Investigations May Be Misleading 137
Gregory S. Finucane

25 New Type of Paroxysmal Events in a Patient with Epilepsy and Learning Difficulties 141
Maria (Meritxell) Oto

26 Is Less Really More? The Pitfalls of an Ambitiously Healthy Diet 147
Marion Lautenschlager

Part V Metabolic Disorders and Autoimmune Encephalopathies

27 Neurometabolic Conditions May Coexist with Symptoms of Autism 157
Susan Byrne and Tammy Hedderly

28 With the Help of a German Dermatologist 161
Josef Priller

29 A Musician Presents with Unusual Facial Movements, Insomnia, and Depression 167
Mark Groves

30 The Division Between Psychiatric and Neurological Practice Does Not Help Patients with Disorders That Span the Two 171
Belinda Lennox

31 First-Episode Psychosis with Autoimmune Antibodies Involving Clear Neuropsychological Impairment with Common and Unusual Features 175
Patrick Vesey, Paul Maddison, Eileen Ellen T. O'Regan, and Eleanor Williams

32 Subacute Onset of Psychosis with Epileptic Seizures and Dysautonomia: Think Autoimmunity! 181
Til Menge, Diamandis Toutzaris, and Rüdiger J. Seitz

33 Case Study: Anti-GAD Encephalitis 185
Helen Walker, Ashwani Jha, Paul Holmes, Thomasin Andrews, Michael Kopelman, and Mervi Pitkanen

Part VI Organic Psychosis and Organic Personality Disorders

34 Animals in My Tummy 193
Fernando Lázaro Perlado

35 Personality Changes After Encephalitis: When "Organic Personality Disorder" Is Not Enough 199
Maria del Mar Amador and Thomas Mauras

36 Case Vignette. Brain Injury Can Make One Better! 207
Kanu Achinivu

Part VII Other Neuropsychiatric Disorders

37 Psychosis Following Traumatic Brain Injury 213
Tarek Zghoul and Kieran O'Driscoll

38 Bilateral Lesions of the Thalamus: A Neuropsychiatric Challenge 217
Lars Wojtecki and Alfons Schnitzler

39 Listening to the Music and the Patient 223
Jan Adriaan Coebergh

40 Autistic Disorder in Neurofibromatosis 227
Stefanie C. Linden

41 Case Vignette: When You Can't Make Sense of the Story 231
Hilary Lloyd

Contributors

Kanu Achinivu, MBBS, MSc, MRCPsych Department of Neuropsychiatry, National Centre for Mental Health, The Barberry, Birmingham, UK

Thomasin Andrews, BSc, MD, FRCP Department of Neurology, Guy's and St Thomas' NHS Foundation Trust, St Thomas' Hospital, London, UK

Marlies Baldee-Hordijk, MD Centre for Mental Health Care Delfland, Delft, The Netherlands

Roger A. Barker, BA, MBBS, MRCP, PhD John van Geest Centre for Brain Repair, Addenbrooke's Hospital, Cambridge, UK

Frank Besag, BSc, MSc, PhD, MBChB East London NHS Foundation Trust, Mid Bedfordshire Clinic, Bedford, UK

Christopher R. Butler, MA, MRCP, PhD Department of Clinical Neurosciences, John Radcliffe Hospital, Oxford, UK

Susan Byrne, MB, BAO, BCh, PhD, MRCPI, MRCPCH Paediatric Neurology, Evelina Children's Hospital, St. Thomas' Hospital, London, UK

Andrea E. Cavanna, MD, PhD Department of Neuropsychiatry, The Barberry National Centre for Mental Health, Birmingham, UK

Jan Adriaan Coebergh, MBBS, FRCP Department of Neurology, Ashford St Peter's Foundation NHS Trust, Chertsey, UK

Gemma Cummins, MB, MRCPI John van Geest Centre for Brain Repair, Addenbrooke's Hospital, Cambridge, UK

M. A. J. de Koning-Tijssen, MD, PhD Department of Neurology, University Medical Center Groningen, Groningen, The Netherlands

Maria del Mar Amador, MD Départemente de Neurologie, Groupe Hospitalier Pitié-Salpétriêre, Paris, France

Emma Devenney, MB, BCh, BAO, MRCP Neuroscience Research Australia, Sydney, NSW, Australia

Valsamma Eapen, MBBS, PhD, FRCPsych, FRANZCP Academic Unit of Child Psychiatry South West Sydney (AUCS), School of Psychiatry, Mental Health Centre, Liverpool Hospital, University of New South Wales and Liverpool Hospital, Sydney, NSW, Australia

Mark J. Edwards, PhD Institute of Cardiovascular and Cell Sciences, St. George's University of London, London, UK

Gregory S. Finucane, MBChB, MA, FRANZCP Auckland City Hospital, Auckland, New Zealand

K. Foy, MB, BCh, BAO, MSc, MRCPI, MRCPsych The Walton Centre NHS Foundation Trust, Liverpool, UK

J. M. Gelauff, MD Department of Neurology, University Medical Center Groningen, Groningen, The Netherlands

Harald Gelderblom, MD Abteilung Medizin, GKV-Spitzenverband, Berlin, Germany

Mark Groves, MD Department of Psychiatry, Icahn School of Medicine at Mt. Sinai, New York, NY, USA

Tammy Hedderly, MBBS, BSc (Hons), FRPCH Evelina London Children's Hospital and St Thomas' Hospital, London, UK

John Hodges, MBBS, FRCPF, MedSci, FRACP Neuroscience Research Australia, Sydney, NSW, Australia

Paul Holmes, MD, FRCP (UK) Department of Neurology, Guy's and St Thomas' NHS Foundation Trust, St Thomas' Hospital, London, UK

Martin Holtkamp, MD Department of Neurology, Epilepsy-Center Berlin-Brandenburg, Charité – Universitätsmedizin Berlin, Berlin, Germany

Ashwani Jha, MRCP, PhD Department of Neurology, St Thomas' Hospital, London, UK

Michael Kopelman, PhD, FBPsS, FRCPsych, FMedSci Department of Academic Neuropsychiatry, King's College London, St Thomas's Hospital, London, UK

Marion Lautenschlager, MD, Dipl Chem Department of Neuropsychiatry, Charité – Universitätsmedizin Berlin, Berlin, Germany

James F. Leckman, MD, PhD Yale School of Medicine, Child Study Center, New Haven, CT, USA

Teresa Lee, BA (Hons), M Psychol, PhD Neuropsychiatric Institute, Prince of Wales Hospital, NPI, Euroa Centre, Sydney, NSW, Australia

Belinda Lennox, BMedSci, BM, BS, MRCPsych Department of Psychiatry, University of Oxford, Warneford Hospital, Headington, Oxford, UK

Stefanie C. Linden, MD, PhD Institute of Psychological Medicine and Clinical Neurosciences, Cardiff University School of Medicine, Cardiff, UK

Hilary Lloyd, MB, ChB, FRCPsych Child & Adolescent Mental Health Services, Royal Manchester Children's Hospital, Manchester, UK

Paul Maddison, MD, FRCP Department of Neurology, Queen's Medical Centre, Nottingham, UK

Thomas Mauras, MD Service de Psychiatrie, Institut Hospitalo-Universitaire de l'Institut du Cerveau et de la Moelle Epinière, Groupe Hospitalier Pitié-Salpétriêre, Paris, France

Ian McKeith, MD, FRCPsych, FRSB, FMedSci Institute for Ageing, Newcastle University, Newcastle upon Tyne, UK

Til Menge, MD Department of Neurology, LVR-Klinikum Düsseldorf, Heinrich-Heine-University Düsseldorf, Düsseldorf, Germany

Adith Mohan, MBBS, MRCPsych, FRANZCP Neuropsychiatric Institute, Prince of Wales Hospital, NPI, Euroa Centre, Sydney, NSW, Australia

Kieran O'Driscoll, FRCPsych David Lewis Centre, Cheshire, UK

Eileen Ellen T. O'Regan, MB, BCh, BAO, MRCPsych Marlow House, Early Intervention in Psychosis Service, Nottingham, UK

Maria (Meritxell) Oto, LGMS, PhD, MECPsych Department of Neuropsychiatry, Scottish Epilepsy Centre, Glasgow, UK

Fernando Lázaro Perlado, LMS, MSc, MRCPsych Department of Neuropsychiatry, R.S.M.B. Hospital de Bermeo, Bermeo, Bizkaia, Spain

Clínica Indautxu, Bilbao, Bizkaia, Spain

Mervi Pitkanen, MBBS, Lic Med, MA, MRC Psych, MD Department of Neuropsychiatry and Memory Disorders, King's College London, London, UK

Josef Priller, MD Department of Neuropsychiatry, Charité – Universitätsmedizin Berlin, Berlin, Germany

Hugh Rickards, MBChB, MD, FRCPsych, MMedSci Department of Neuropsychiatry, Birmingham University Birmingham and Solihull Mental Health Foundation Trust, Birmingham, UK

Renata Rizzo, MD, PhD Department of Medical and Pediatric Science, Azienda Policlinico-OVE, Catania University, Catania, Italy

Mary May Robertson, MB, MD, DSc, FRCPCH, FRCP, FRCPsych Emeritus (University College London), London, UK

Honorary University Cape Town, Cape Town, South Africa

St Georges Hospital, London, UK

Perminder Sachdev, MBBS, MD, PhD, FRANZCP Neuropsychiatric Institute, Prince of Wales Hospital, NPI, Euroa Centre, Sydney, NSW, Australia

Alfons Schnitzler, MD Department of Neurology, and Institute of Clinical Neuroscience and Medical Psychology, Universitätsklinikum Duesseldorf, Düsseldorf, Germany

Rüdiger J. Seitz, MD Department of Neurology, LVR-Klinikum Düsseldorf, Heinrich-Heine-University Düsseldorf, Düsseldorf, Germany

Hugh Selsick, MBBCh, BSC (Hon) University College London Hospitals, Insomnia Clinic, Royal London Hospital for Integrated Medicine, London, UK

Eike Jakob Spruth, MD Department of Neuropsychiatry, Charité – Universitätsmedizin Berlin, Berlin, Germany

Jon Stone, MB, ChB, FRCP, PhD Department of Clinical Neurosciences, University of Edinburgh, Western General Hospital, Edinburgh, UK

Tillmann Supprian, MD, PhD Section of Geriatric Psychiatry, Department of Psychiatry and Psychotherapy, Medical Faculty, Heinrich-Heine University, Düsseldorf, Germany

Tiago Teodoro, MD Institute of Cardiovascular and Cell Sciences, St. George's University of London, London, UK

Department of Neurosciences, Hospital de Santa Maria, Lisbon, Portugal

Instituto de Medicina Molecular, Lisbon, Portugal

Diamandis Toutzaris, MD Department of Neurology, LVR-Klinikum Düsseldorf, Heinrich-Heine-University Düsseldorf, Düsseldorf, Germany

Erik van Duijn, MD, PhD Centre for Mental Health Care Delfland, Leiden University Medical Centre, Delft, The Netherlands

Patrick Vesey, BSc (Hons), D Clin Psych Department of Clinical Psychology and Neuropsychology, Nottingham University Hospitals NHS Trust, Queen's Medical Centre, Nottingham, UK

Helen Walker, MBChB, MRCPsych Department of Neuropsychiatry, St Thomas's Hospital, London, UK

Killian Welch, MBChB, MPhil, MD Robert Fergusson Unit, Royal Edinburgh Hospital, Edinburgh, UK

Eleanor Williams, BSc, MSc Department of Clinical and Neuropsychology, Nottingham University Hospitals NHS Trust, Queen's Medical Centre, Nottingham, UK

Lars Wojtecki, MD Department of Neurology, Institute of Clinical Neuroscience and Medical Psychology, Universitätsklinikum Düsseldorf, Düsseldorf, Germany

Adam Zeman, BA, BM, BCh, DM, FRCP Cognitive and Behavioural Neurology, University of Exeter Medical School, Exeter, UK

Tarek Zghoul, MBChB, PhD Department of Psychiatry, Oxford University, Warneford Hospital, Oxford, UK

Part I
Dementias

Chapter 1
Unexplained Delirium, Atypical Dementia, and Prodromal DLB

Ian McKeith

In 1982, I was asked by a general practitioner to urgently see a 72-year-old man who earlier that day had tried to break down a door at the back of his house in order to escape a perceived intrusion by armed men. It was our habit then to see most new psychiatric referrals at home typically accompanied by medical students who enjoyed escaping the hospital for a ride in my car.

His wife told me that her husband had not been himself since retirement from a manual job 5 years earlier. Never a talkative man, he had become increasingly quiet and withdrawn with little interest in his garden or other activities. He had also become physically slower and spent several hours a day sleeping in his chair if left undisturbed. His wife wondered if he was depressed, but since he made no complaints and his mood did not seem low, they sought no help at that stage.

For the last year, he had started to have episodes of confusion in which he appeared not to be fully orientated and spoke about seeing people in his house when his wife was clear that nobody was there. In between these episodes, he was more forgetful than previously although this was variable and at times he seemed almost his normal self. Over the last 2 months, he had repeatedly talked about seeing soldiers hiding in the rosebushes in his garden. These frightened him, and it was in response to thinking that they were about to come into his house and shoot him and his wife that he made the escape attempt that led to my visit. When asked if the soldiers were still there, he pulled aside the lace curtains from across the windows and pointed at the bushes but said that they had gone. He seemed to have partial insight that they might not have been real and agreed that his eyes might have been playing a trick on him.

My notes on the day recorded a slow-moving, slightly stooped man with a fixed and slightly gloomy facial expression and gaze which I judged to represent a mild clouding of consciousness. He was slow to answer questions, scoring 20/30 on the

I. McKeith, MD, FRC Psych, FRSB, F Med Sci
Institute for Ageing, Newcastle University, Newcastle upon Tyne, UK
e-mail: i.g.mckeith@ncl.ac.uk

J. Priller, H. Rickards (eds.), *Neuropsychiatry Case Studies*,
DOI 10.1007/978-3-319-42190-2_1

mini-mental state examination (MMSE) and completely unable to copy a pentagon or subtract serial sevens but recalling two out of three objects and all three with cueing. He had a slightly flexed posture on walking which could be taken as normal for age but no other parkinsonian features.

My preferred diagnosis was a delirium of uncertain etiology in a man with possible early dementia, occurring in the setting of a postretirement chronic depression. In view of his vivid and complex visual hallucinations, I recommended haloperidol 1 mg tds and arranged investigation of the cause of his delirium at a day hospital. Midstream specimen of urine (MSU), routine bloods, and physical examination revealed no significant abnormalities, but his general condition was noted to be deteriorating very quickly with rigidity, immobility, and failure to eat and drink. He died suddenly after a large hematemesis within 2 weeks of the initial referral.

His diagnosis remained a mystery, and he was considered then to be one of a group of patients who we saw with "atypical" dementia associated with delirium and a poor prognosis.

Because there was an active dementia research program in the hospital where I was working, it was fairly routine to ask for neuropathological autopsy which we extended to these "atypical" cases. This showed that in addition to mild plaque and tangle Alzheimer pathology, this patient also had extensive cortical Lewy bodies. He therefore fell into a diagnostic category of senile dementia of the Lewy body type (SDLT), the first of a series of 21 such cases that we had seen at autopsy by 1990 and which others were also beginning to describe elsewhere around the world. Three stages of illness were proposed with the first stage being "usually recognized only in retrospect and extending back 1–3 years pre-presentation with occasional minor episodes of forgetfulness sometimes described as lapses of concentration or 'switching off'. A brief period of delirium was sometimes noted for the first time in association with genuine physical illness and/or surgical procedures but was followed by full recovery and did not prompt psychiatric referral. Patients were subsequently able to function adequately in activities of daily living although relatives and carers reported a subsequent mental and physical decline" [1].

If the same patient was referred to me today, I hope that the diagnosis of dementia with Lewy bodies (DLB) would have been suspected at first visit due to the combination of all three core features of the disorder, namely, cognitive fluctuation, recurrent visual hallucinations, and parkinsonism (Table 1.1). Also typical was the apathy, daytime drowsiness, and the cognitive profile with differentially impaired visuospatial task performance and relatively preserved memory. I would now ask routinely after a history of REM sleep behavior disorder (RBD) which is typical, often preceding other symptoms by up to a decade and which is rare in other dementing disorders. Investigation would still include a search for precipitants for the delirious features but would recognize that these can occur spontaneously in DLB without external provocation. Haloperidol or indeed any antipsychotic medications should be avoided because of the known sensitivity of DLB patients to dopaminergic blockade, with a two- to threefold increased mortality. Management would center on a combination of explanation and reassurance, manipulation of the precipitating environment, and the use of cholinesterase inhibitors. Removing the lace curtains and digging up the rosebushes might be part of the treatment plan.

Table 1.1 Revised criteria for the clinical diagnosis of dementia with Lewy bodies (DLB) [2]

1. *Central feature* (essential for a diagnosis of possible or probable DLB)
Dementia defined as progressive cognitive decline of sufficient magnitude to interfere with normal social or occupational function
Prominent or persistent memory impairment may not necessarily occur in the early stages but is usually evident with progression
Deficits on tests of attention, executive function, and visuospatial ability may be especially prominent
2. *Core features* (two core features are sufficient for a diagnosis of probable DLB, one for possible DLB)
Fluctuating cognition with pronounced variations in attention and alertness
Recurrent visual hallucinations that are typically well formed and detailed
Spontaneous features of parkinsonism
3. *Suggestive features* (if one or more of these are present in the presence of one or more core features, a diagnosis of probable DLB can be made. In the absence of any core features, one or more suggestive features are sufficient for possible DLB. Probable DLB should not be diagnosed on the basis of suggestive features alone)
REM sleep behavior disorder
Severe neuroleptic sensitivity
Low dopamine transporter uptake in basal ganglia demonstrated by single-photon emission computed tomography (SPECT) or positron emission tomography (PET) imaging
4. *Supportive features* (*commonly present but not proven to have diagnostic specificity*)
Repeated falls and syncope
Transient, unexplained loss of consciousness
Severe autonomic dysfunction, e.g., orthostatic hypotension, urinary incontinence
Hallucinations in other modalities
Systematized delusions
Depression
Relative preservation of medial temporal lobe structures on CT/MRI scan
Generalized low uptake on SPECT/PET perfusion scan with reduced occipital activity
Abnormal (low uptake) metaiodobenzylguanidine (MIBG) myocardial scintigraphy
Prominent slow wave activity on electroencephalogram (EEG) with temporal lobe transient sharp waves
5. *A diagnosis of DLB is less likely*
In the presence of cerebrovascular disease evident as focal neurologic signs or on brain imaging
In the presence of any other physical illness or brain disorder sufficient to account in part or in total for the clinical picture
If parkinsonism only appears for the first time at a stage of severe dementia
6. *Temporal sequence of symptoms*
DLB should be diagnosed when dementia occurs before or concurrently with parkinsonism (if it is present). The term Parkinson disease dementia (PDD) should be used to describe dementia that occurs in the context of well-established Parkinson disease. In a practice setting, the term that is most appropriate to the clinical situation should be used and generic terms such as LB disease are often helpful. In research studies in which distinction needs to be made between DLB and PDD, the existing 1-year rule between the onset of dementia and parkinsonism DLB continues to be recommended. Adoption of other time periods will simply confound data pooling or comparison between studies. In other research settings that may include clinicopathologic studies and clinical trials, both clinical phenotypes may be considered collectively under categories such as LB disease or alpha-synucleinopathy

As dementia syndromes present earlier for diagnosis, DLB often, although not always, comes to attention at a stage when the core features are barely evident. Identifying early or prodromal DLB is a more difficult task and one which has not yet been adequately addressed in diagnostic guidelines and criteria. But we do know that patients with mild non-amnestic cognitive impairments are at particular risk of progression to DLB, especially if they have additional evidence of delirium-like features including cognitive fluctuation and daytime sleepiness [3]. Such cases may meet the currently underused diagnostic category of possible DLB (one core or one suggestive feature only), and it is in this group that demonstration of reduced dopamine transporter uptake in the striatum is a particularly useful diagnostic biomarker, strongly indicative of underlying Lewy body pathology. A normal scan does not however rule out LB disease [4].

DLB patients may also present with acute unexplained or provoked delirium in the general medical clinic, emergency room, and primary care where the index of suspicion for LB disease is low, but the risk of being treated with antipsychotic medication as part of the general management is high.

What Is to Be Learned from This Case?

Firstly, that our diagnostic processes for dementia subtypes have improved over the last 30 years and that any specialist practitioner would now expect to correctly diagnose DLB as presented by my original patient. But the sting in the tail of DLB is that for every one typical case, there are probably at least as many whose clinical presentations are atypical and who are difficult to diagnose even as the disease progresses. This is because the core features may either be absent, e.g., parkinsonism never occurs in 20 % of cases, or the presentation is heavily modified by the presence of concomitant Alzheimer pathology. Clinical diagnosis may therefore range from Alzheimer's disease (the most common misdiagnosis) to vascular dementia (fluctuation, falls, and funny turns) and multisystem atrophy (falls and cognitive decline). So the concepts of "atypical dementia" and "unexplained delirium" remain useful signposts toward DLB as a possible underlying cause. Treatment with cholinesterase inhibitors can be very beneficial and long lasting in DLB and antipsychotics although hazardous, sometimes cannot be avoided, and have to be used with very close monitoring.

References

1. McKeith IG, Perry RH, Fairbairn AF, Jabeen S, Perry EK. Operational criteria for senile dementia of Lewy body type. Psychol Med. 1992;22(4):911–22.
2. McKeith IG, Dickson DW, Lowe J, Emre M, O'Brien JT, Feldman H, et al. Diagnosis and management of dementia with Lewy bodies third report of the DLB consortium. Neurology. 2005;65(12):1863–72.
3. Ferman TJ, Smith GE, Kantarci K, Boeve BF, Pankratz VS, Dickson DW, Dickson DW, et al. Nonamnestic mild cognitive impairment progresses to dementia with Lewy bodies. Neurology. 2013;81(23):2032–8.
4. O'Brien JT, McKeith IG, Walker Z, et al. Diagnostic accuracy of I-123-FP-CIT SPECT in possible dementia with Lewy bodies. Br J Psychiatry. 2009;194(1):34–9.

Chapter 2
Unable to Talk

Fernando Lázaro Perlado

M.A.R. is a 59-year-old female clerical officer who was referred to our clinic as she presented with an anomic aphasia which worsened over the past 3 years, affecting her capacity to communicate and interact with other people, also preventing her from completing her duties. She described her difficulty as being unable to express herself, described word-finding difficulties, as if she had the words she wanted to say "in the tip of her tongue," but unable to say them. There was no other neurological sign nor symptom reported, and except for increased levels of anxiety, she made no other complaint. There was no evidence to support an affective or psychotic disorder.

Background History

She was born from a normal delivery achieving normal developmental milestones. Her childhood and upbringing were uneventful. She completed secondary education after which she started working as a clerical officer. She was described as strong willed and somewhat anxious (a family trait). She never married, currently living with her older brother. She had no psychiatric history of note. She suffered from rheumatoid arthritis, gastroesophageal reflux disease, postmenopausal osteopenia, a successfully removed malignant melanoma (7 years previously), and a mild ferropenic anemia. There was no significant family history.

F. Lázaro Perlado, LMS, MSc, MRCPsych
Department of Neuropsychiatry, R.S.M.B. Hospital de Bermeo, Bermeo, Bizkaia, Spain

Clínica Indautxu, Bilbao, Bizkaia, Spain
e-mail: fernando.lazaroperlado@osakidetza.eus; drflazaro@movistar.es

J. Priller, H. Rickards (eds.), *Neuropsychiatry Case Studies*, DOI 10.1007/978-3-319-42190-2_2

Examination

It revealed a middle-aged Caucasian female smartly dressed and well groomed. She was cooperative. She came across as euthymic with an appropriate affect. Her speech was patently anomic with phonemic and semantic paraphasias and nearly agrammatical. She was able to repeat single words, but not always sentences. She appeared quite anxious during cognitive testing. There was no evidence of any affective or psychotic disorder. In her thought content, she was worried about her speech difficulties and how this affected her capacity to relate to her peers and significant others as well as her inability to meet her job requirements. She showed insight into her predicament.

Bedside Cognitive Testing

She was anxious throughout the testing. She scored 14/30 in the MMSE and 28/100 in the ACEve (Spanish version of the Addenbrooke's Cognitive Examination) although she very well underachieved due to her aphasia. Nevertheless, we could observe problems in her verbal and semantic memory, naming, verbal fluency, attention and concentration, inability to follow complex commands, and inability to repeat sentences, and she showed constructional dyspraxia. She was unable to complete Luria's test, alternate hand movements, and the "go-no go" test. She could not explain any of the three well-known proverbs.

Third Party Information

She is independent in her basic ADLs, but showed some problems in the instrumental ADLs. Her brother also described attention (left the cooker on once or twice) and memory problems (tends to prepare the same meals, forgets recipes having to ring her cousin for advice), inability to do the weekly shopping (being able to buy the odd item), some difficulties in administering her monies, a self-imposed allowance, and an increase in her alcohol consumption not reaching misuse or dependency levels.

Investigations

1. Blood screening:
   Only detected mildly elevated cholesterol and a mild ferropenic anemia. VDRL and HIV testing were negative.
2. Brain MRI:
   (a) December 2012:
   It detected a discrete enlargement of the ventricular system and cerebral sulci to correlate with the adequate clinical picture. Microinfarcts can be seen in

the subcortical white matter in no significant number to the patient's age and none acute or hemorrhagic. No other significant abnormalities.

(b) February 2014:
It detected hyperintensities in the periventricular white matter suggestive of periventricular ischemic leukopathy. It also showed small bilateral hyperintensities within the frontal white matter of probable ischemic origin. The cisterns, ventricles, and sulci are prominent, reflecting a degree of brain atrophy. The vascular system is of normal morphology. No sellar or parasellar abnormalities detected.

3. Brain SPECT, May 2014:
It detected a heterogeneous pattern of hypoperfusion in the left cerebral hemisphere, more prominent in the parietal cortex and the superior frontal and temporal cortices, and a very mild hypoperfusion in the left thalamus and the right parietal cortex.

4. Neuropsychometry:
Detected a severe language impairment which affects expression, naming, writing, and to a lesser extent repetition. It also detected a mild to moderate impairment in working memory, memory fixation, calculus, praxias, and abstract verbal reasoning.
Its functional impact is discrete, but difficulties administering money and some abnormal behaviors are starting to emerge.
The neuropsychologist concluded that her findings were compatible with a neurodegenerative process not only limited to a language dysfunction.

Summary

The more striking feature of this patient's clinical presentation is the language problem with a patent anomic aphasia, but also naming, repetition, and comprehension problems. It started some 3 years before, showing a more pronounced deterioration during the 6–9 months prior to our review. Bedside cognitive testing, allowing of her language problem, detected a wider cognitive dysfunction affecting other cognitive domains. It made us request a detailed neuropsychometric assessment as we felt that a more generalized cognitive impairment was present underneath the anomic aphasia.

Structural neuroimaging showed a generalized brain atrophy (no specific hippocampal analysis was performed) with minor ischemic changes that wouldn't stand to explain the clinical picture (Figs. 2.1 and 2.2).

Functional neuroimaging showed hypoperfusion to both parietal cortices, more prominent in the left hemisphere, and also to the superior left frontal and temporal cortices (Fig. 2.3).

Differential Diagnosis

Our patient fulfills the core clinical criteria for all-cause dementia [1] presenting cognitive symptoms that interfere with her ability to work and her usual activities, represent a decline from previous level of functioning, and are not explained by

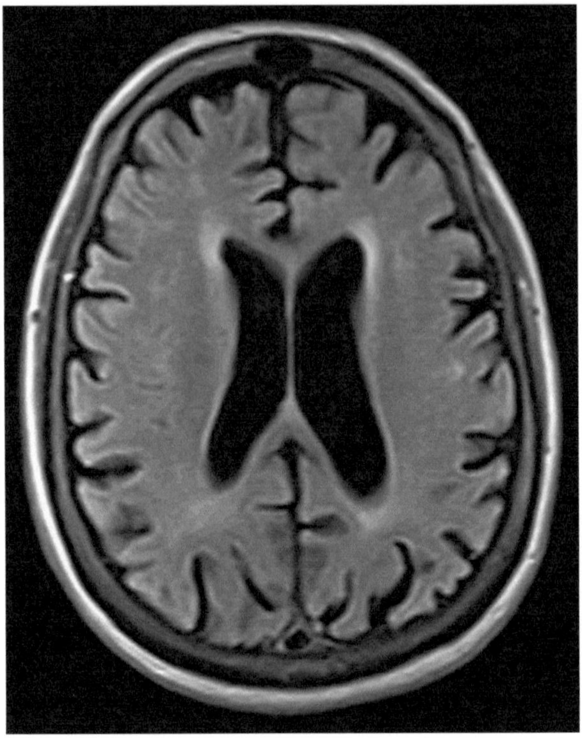

Fig. 2.1 Axial cranial MRI, T1 sequence, showing a mild to moderate generalized atrophy with periventricular hyperintensities as well as small juxtacortical ones

delirium or major psychiatric disorder; the cognitive impairment is diagnosed objectively and involves various cognitive domains (impaired ability to acquire new information, visuospatial abilities, language, and reasoning abilities).

With this in mind, the main diagnostic categories to consider in this case would be:

1. Multi-infarct dementia:
   Although the MRIs have detected ischemic lesions (hyperintensities in T2) (Fig. 2.1), these are not big enough nor numerous enough to be responsible for this lady's problems. Moreover, there is no temporal relationship between the onset of the language difficulties and clear ischemic lesions on MRI. In fact, in order to assume that small vessel disease is the cause of vascular cognitive impairment, hyperintensities affecting at least a quarter of the white matter are needed.
2. Nonfluent primary progressive aphasia:
   Although in our patient the more prominent clinical feature is difficulty in language, with naming, writing, and comprehension problems, there are other cognitive domains also affected. Besides, the neuroimaging findings – both structural and functional – do not support this. Abnormalities in the left posterior fronto-insular region and supplementary motor areas and inferior frontal gyrus (Broca's area) are necessary for an imaging-supported diagnosis. In this case, there is a generalized cerebral atrophy.

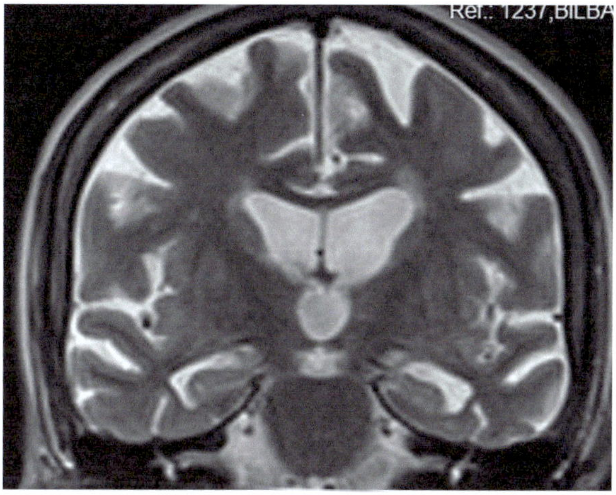

Fig. 2.2 Coronal cranial MRI, T2 sequence, showing moderate generalized brain atrophy together with periventricular and juxtacortical hyperintensities

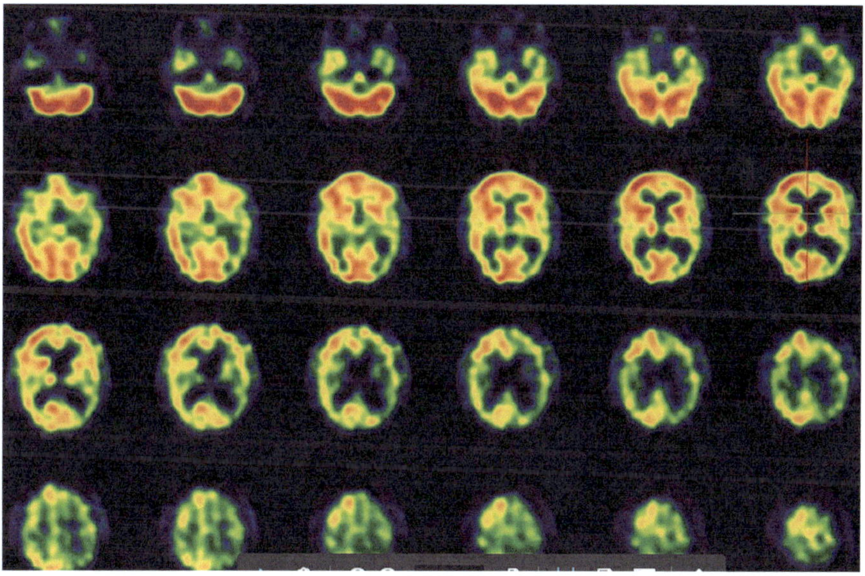

Fig. 2.3 Cerebral SPECT, axial view, showing a heterogeneous pattern of hypoperfusion in the left cerebral hemisphere

3. Logopenic progressive aphasia:
   The more recently described subtype of PPA, and consistently associated with Alzheimer's disease (AD), is defined by impaired naming and sentence repetition with preservation of grammar and motor aspects of speech. By definition, there is preservation of semantic knowledge [2].
   Our patient presented with naming difficulties and sentence repetition, but also with semantic memory problems. She also showed inability to follow complex commands, perhaps reflecting executive problems to be expected in a case of AD.

4. Atypical presentation of Alzheimer's disease [3, 4]:
   In this particular case, the patient presents with an anomic aphasia with cognitive difficulties encompassing other cognitive domains. Structural neuroimaging shows generalized brain atrophy, and the SPECT pattern of perfusion is not compatible with PPA. A nonfluent aphasia has been described as an atypical form of presentation of AD.
   Although diagnostic certainty will only be ascertained postmortem, and although we accept the possibility of a mixed etiology (vascular/AD), our view is that, in our patient, an atypical presentation of AD could very well be the case.

Learning Points

One must not assume a diagnosis without in-depth assessment and investigation.

- In this case, an in-depth neuropsychological assessment detected other cognitive problems.
- Structural and functional neuroimaging is also pointed toward a mixed/AD dementia [5].

References

1. McKhan MG, Knopman DS, Chertkow H, et al. The diagnosis of dementia due to Alzheimer's disease: recommendations from the National Institute on Aging-Alzheimer's Association workgroups on diagnostic guidelines for Alzheimer's disease. Alzheimers Dement. 2011;7: 263–9.
2. Leyton CE, Piguet O, Savage S, Burrell J, Hodges JR. The neural basis of logopenic progressive aphasia. J Alzheimers Dis. 2012;32:1051–9.
3. Galton CJ, Patterson K, Xuereb JH, Hodges JR. Atypical and typical presentations of Alzheimer's disease: a clinical, neuropsychological, neuroimaging and pathological study of 13 cases. Brain. 2000;123:484–98.
4. Gorno-Tempini ML, Hillis AE, Weintraub S, et al. Classification of primary progressive aphasia and its variants. Neurology. 2011;76:1006–14.
5. Harper L, Barkhof F, Scheltens P, Schott JM, Fox NC. An algorithmic approach to structural imaging in dementia. J Neurol Neurosurg Psychiatry. 2014;85:692–8.

Chapter 3
A Mistaken Recurrent Depression

Eike Jakob Spruth

EE, a 75-year-old retired primary school teacher, was referred to our institution for neuropsychiatric evaluation with an approximately 1-year history of depressed mood and mental overload. Over the course of time, she had experienced alternating episodes of paranoid and nihilistic delusions with stupor. She had been an inpatient on a psychiatric ward for almost 1 year with only two short interruptions of a few weeks. Treatment-resistant depression was diagnosed as several antidepressants (venlafaxine, moclobemide, citalopram, tranylcypromine, phenelzine), lithium, antipsychotic drugs (haloperidol, risperidone, promethazine), and sedatives (lorazepam) had failed despite of high doses.

At admission to our hospital, the patient received haloperidol (5 mg per day), promethazine (25 mg per day), and lorazepam (2 mg per day), furthermore pantoprazole, torasemide, diclofenac, and calcium.

Background History

EE was married and childless. She had suffered from recurrent depression since her retirement at the age of 64 years. She incurred about two major depressive episodes per year. A cognitive testing performed 18 months before the present admission had shown no significant impairment. Six months ago, spatial disorientation and visuospatial deficits on the clock-drawing test were revealed but attributed to the mood disorder.

Examination

EE was awake and fully oriented to person, place, time, and situation. She answered questions with long latencies. Her mood was depressed, her affect was blunted, and she showed severely impaired motivation. Nihilistic delusions were present. In the mini-mental state examination, she achieved a score of 24 out of 30 (amnestic

E.J. Spruth, MD
Department of Neuropsychiatry, Charité – Universitätsmedizin Berlin, Berlin, Germany
e-mail: eike.spruth@charite.de

J. Priller, H. Rickards (eds.), *Neuropsychiatry Case Studies*,
DOI 10.1007/978-3-319-42190-2_3

deficits, dyscalculia, visuospatial deficits). Her Hamilton Depression Rating Scale (HAMD) score was 30.

The neurological examination revealed parkinsonism with hypokinesia and muscular rigidity.

Initial Investigations

Routine MRI showed low-grade microangiopathy without significant atrophy. The EEG was normal. Routine blood screening did not reveal any clinically significant abnormalities. The screening for malignancies or autoimmune disease was negative.

Differential Diagnosis

As the patient had a known history of recurrent depression, we initially assumed that EE suffered from a major depressive episode with psychotic features. However, unlike former episodes, this depressive episode was resistant to antidepressant treatment, and, in addition, EE showed signs of cognitive impairment.

Further Investigation

We performed a lumbar puncture, which revealed increased tau protein and a decreased beta-amyloid ratio ($A\beta_{1-42}/A\beta_{1-40}$ ratio = 0.03) in the CSF. The patient also received an FDG-PET (with 271 MBq F^{18}-FDG), which showed moderately reduced tracer uptake in the right inferior temporolateral cortex and in the posterior cingulum/precuneus and the parietotemporal cortex bilaterally (Fig. 3.1).

Diagnosis

Based on the clinical findings, the results of the CSF analysis, and the FDG-PET, we diagnosed an organic affective disorder as a consequence of Alzheimer's disease (AD) in EE.

Progress

We discontinued haloperidol and promethazine and tapered off lorazepam, resulting in a complete remission of the Parkinsonism, an increase in motivation, and a normalization of cognitive speed. Next, we treated EE with donepezil, which may improve

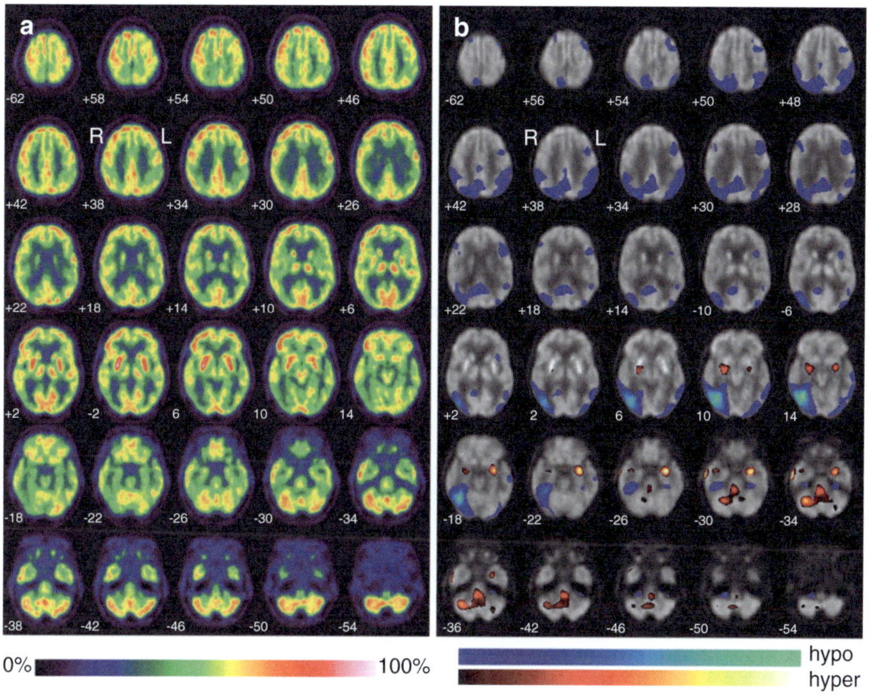

Fig. 3.1 The FDG-PET (**a**) reveals significant hypometabolism in the temporoparietal cortex based on pattern recognition at $p<0.01$ (**b**)

not only cognitive but also neuropsychiatric symptoms of AD [1]. The delusions successively diminished concomitant with an improvement of mood. When EE was discharged from our hospital at 10 weeks after admission, she scored 4 in the HAMD.

What Did I Learn from This Case?

Depression is common in the early stages of AD [2, 3] and may even be a harbinger of future cognitive decline in cognitively healthy older subjects [4]. Masters et al. [5] recently described depression as part of the initial phase of "noncognitive" AD.

In our case, dementia presented with symptoms of a major depression 1 year before significant cognitive decline, which is why the neuropsychiatric symptoms were mistaken for a primary psychiatric disorder. Cognitive impairment as well as affective symptoms in the elderly requires thorough differential diagnostic consideration of both a major depressive episode and early forms of dementia.

References

1. Cummings JL, Mackell J, Kaufer D. Behavioral effects of current Alzheimer's disease treatments: a descriptive review. Alzheimers Dement. 2008;4(1):49–60.

2. Ismail Z, Smith EE, Geda Y, Sultzer D, Brodaty H, Smith G, Aguera-Ortiz L, Sweet R, Miller D, Lyketsos CG, ISTAART Neuropsychiatric Symptoms Professional Interest Area. Neuropsychiatric symptoms as early manifestations of emergent dementia: provisional diagnostic criteria for mild behavioral impairment. Alzheimers Dement. 2016;12(2):195–202.
3. Woolley JD, Khan BK, Murthy NK, Miller BL, Rankin KP. The diagnostic challenge of psychiatric symptoms in neurodegenerative disease: rates of and risk factors for prior psychiatric diagnosis in patients with early neurodegenerative disease. J Clin Psychiatry. 2011;72(2):126–33.
4. Banks SJ, Raman R, He F, Salmon DP, Ferris S, Aisen P, et al. The Alzheimer's disease cooperative study prevention instrument project: longitudinal outcome of behavioral measures as predictors of cognitive decline. Dement Geriatr Cogn Dis Extra. 2014;4(3):509–16.
5. Masters MC, Morris JC, Roe CM. "Noncognitive" symptoms of early Alzheimer disease: a longitudinal analysis. Neurology. 2015;84(6):617–22.

Chapter 4
An Atypical Variant of a Common Neurodegenerative Disorder

Adith Mohan, Teresa Lee, and Perminder Sachdev

AB is a 62-year-old retired gentleman living with his wife who was referred for diagnostic workup following outpatient review in the neuropsychiatric clinic. There was a 3-year history of progressive deficits in cognitive functioning of insidious onset, and characterized initially by prominent language and visuospatial deficits, with memory impairment noted more recently.

The patient's problems first became apparent 3 years ago, following a motor vehicle accident wherein AB misjudged a kerb when driving and ran over the top of a gutter. Other examples of visuospatial difficulties noted over time included an inability to line up a screwdriver with a nail, something out of character for a man known to be quite proficient with tools, and difficulty in judging stairs resulting in two falls. He was also noted at around the same time to have stopped reading, when he had previously been an avid reader, and his handwriting became less defined and poorer in quality. In the last 12–18 months, he was reported to have significant word-finding difficulties, leading to a restriction in his social repertoire. AB reported a history of social anxiety that was most significant when he was required to have face-to-face conversations, with worsening in speech difficulties during these times.

In the 8–12 months prior to his presentation, AB began to have trouble dressing himself and using cutlery without assistance. He was unable to shave independently, repeatedly cutting himself, and was no longer able to cook meals. Although able to identify the ingredients correctly, he could not work out how to put the meal together.

A. Mohan, MBBS, MRCPsych, FRANZCP • T. Lee, BA (Hons), M Psychol, PhD
P. Sachdev, MBBS, MD, PhD, FRANZCP (✉)
Neuropsychiatric Institute, Prince of Wales Hospital, NPI, Euroa Centre, Sydney, NSW, Australia
e-mail: a.mohan@unsw.edu.au; teresa.lee@unsw.edu.au; p.sachdev@unsw.edu.au

J. Priller, H. Rickards (eds.), *Neuropsychiatry Case Studies*,
DOI 10.1007/978-3-319-42190-2_4

Background History

AB was the middle of three siblings, and there was no history of perinatal insult or developmental deviance. He was premorbidly well adjusted socially and studied to 10 years equivalent in mainstream schooling. He then worked in a hardware store for 18 months and joined the navy at age 17 years, serving in combat during the Vietnam conflict and developing chronic post-traumatic stress disorder (PTSD) as a result, residual symptoms of which had persisted. There was also a 30-year history of alcohol abuse, currently in remission. Psychiatric history was remarkable also for a recurrent depressive disorder with history of attempted suicide by overdose in his early 20s and approximately one to two relapse episodes per year necessitating occasional inpatient psychiatric treatment and long-term maintenance therapy with moclobemide. Previous treatment trials for depression included fluvoxamine, Sertraline, citalopram, desvenlafaxine, amitriptyline, nefazodone, thioridazine, and augmentation with low-dose sodium valproate as a mood stabilizer in addition to previous psychological therapy targeting PTSD and depressive symptomatology. These symptoms resulted in significant marital dysfunction and divorce from his first wife after 15 years of marriage. He had remarried at age 50 years with both AB and his wife reporting their relationship to be stable.

He was an ex-smoker and reported a mild head injury at age 50 years, with no loss of consciousness or neurological or neurocognitive sequelae. There was no reported family history of neurodegenerative or other neurological disorders.

Examination

AB was a Caucasian gentleman of medium build who was cooperative with assessment. There was no evidence of overt psychomotor agitation or obvious involuntary movement disorder. In particular, there was no evidence of parkinsonism, nor were there cerebellar or frontal release signs noted on examination. His speech was fluent but with prominent word-finding pauses, and his affect was labile with episodes of tearfulness (congruent to themes of discussion). He was noted to have impaired left-right orientation, finger agnosia, constructional apraxia, dyscalculia, and bilateral upper limb agraphesthesia. Ocular apraxia was absent, and extraocular movements were full and normal as was his gait. He had partial insight into his cognitive deficits. Detailed neuropsychological assessment was carried out and the results are presented below.

Investigations

Routine blood screening did not show any abnormalities. EEG demonstrated diffuse slowing with delta and theta activity with eyes closed and poorly formed posterior rhythms of 6–7 Hz frequency. MRI demonstrated a few foci of deep white matter hyperintensities on fluid-attenuated inversion recovery (FLAIR) imaging, with no

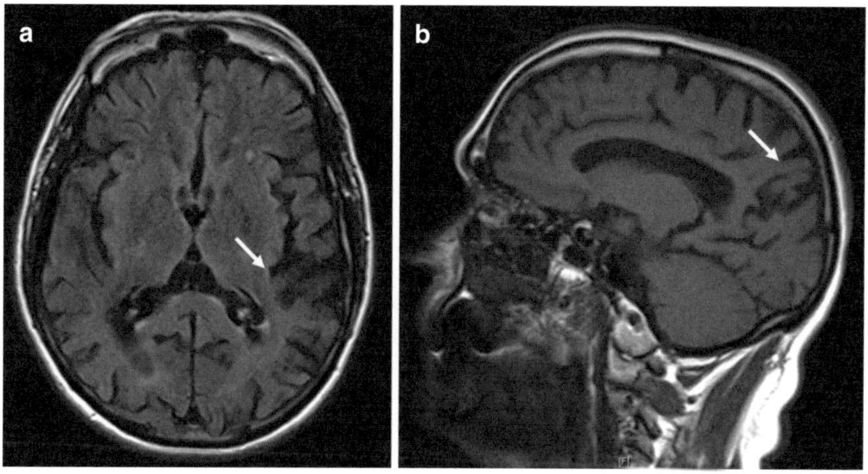

Fig. 4.1 (**a**) T2 FLAIR axial image and (**b**) T1 sagittal image showing prominent parietal atrophy (*arrows*)

abnormal parenchymal signal otherwise seen. Moderate enlargement of the ventricles and CSF spaces in keeping with central and peripheral atrophy was noted. Biparietal atrophy was noted to be relatively prominent (Fig. 4.1). The midline structures including the brainstem, pituitary, and corpus callosum as well as the cerebellum were normal in appearance. Functional imaging with positron emission tomography (PET) using ^{18}F-deoxyglucose showed marked reduction in metabolism in both parietal lobes, more marked on the left.

Neuropsychological Assessment

AB had previously been assessed 24 months ago by another health facility, where he demonstrated widespread cognitive deficits, suggestive of a neurodegenerative process.

When neuropsychological assessment was conducted on this occasion, AB was alert though appearing bewildered. His verbal responses were hesitant, but spontaneous speech was relatively fluent. Some utilization behavior was demonstrated with the objects on the examiner's desk. He had difficulty comprehending the instructions of some tasks despite simplification and repetition, at times being unable to do so. He could not tell the time on his digital watch. He had great difficulty in judging the height of (or distance from) each step and held on to the railing of both sides of the stairs on his way to and from the examiner's office.

On cognitive screening with the Addenbrooke's Cognitive Examination-III [1], AB performed poorly in attention (5/18), memory (7/26), fluency (1/14), and visuospatial (4/16) domains and relatively better in language (17/26). He wrote his name with difficulty, misspelling his first name. He made errors in the most basic tasks of counting forward and backward from "1" to "10" and in reciting the alphabet. He

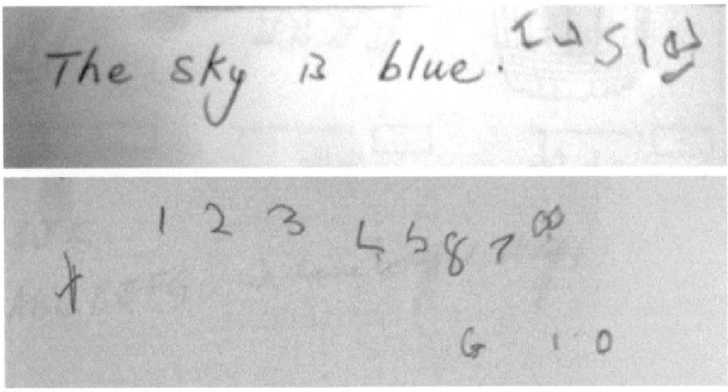

Fig. 4.2 Examples of agraphia (copy a sentence, writing numbers 1–10)

could read single words but not a paragraph. He made spelling mistakes in single word dictation. His writing of some numbers was incomplete, and he could not write a sentence to dictation nor could he copy the same (Fig. 4.2).

On formal cognitive assessment, AB's verbal abstract reasoning ability was borderline impaired, whereas his visuospatial and constructional skills (as shown in a block assembly task) were markedly impaired. His learning and memory of verbal information (a word list) and his visual recognition memory were significantly impaired. His attention and working memory span were limited to being able to repeat three digits forward and two digits backward. Verbal fluency and simple visuospatial planning (clock drawing) were poor, as shown during cognitive screening. He was unable to participate in other measures of executive functions such as cognitive flexibility and response inhibition or tests of psychomotor and processing speed, as he could not comprehend the requirements of these tasks. Regarding parietal functions, AB demonstrated all the features of Gerstmann's syndrome: finger agnosia, acalculia, agraphia, and left-right disorientation. Praxis in the form of pantomime (such as wave goodbye, play the piano) was intact, but constructional dyspraxia was evident (Fig. 4.3).

Further assessment of language functions (at single word level), including picture naming, comprehension, repetition, and semantic association, resulted in a much lower than expected level of performance. Assessment of visual processing (object and space perception) resulted in very poor performance in deciphering incomplete letters, dot counting, object decision, and naming of silhouettes of animals and objects.

When AB's level of performance was compared to his results 2 years ago, further decline was evident in some areas of his already impaired performance, confirming progression over time.

Diagnosis and Differential Diagnosis

The patient's presentation and neuropsychological profile were demonstrative of significant and progressive impairment in language function and visuospatial domain, with his visuospatial processing deficits and parietal dysfunction being

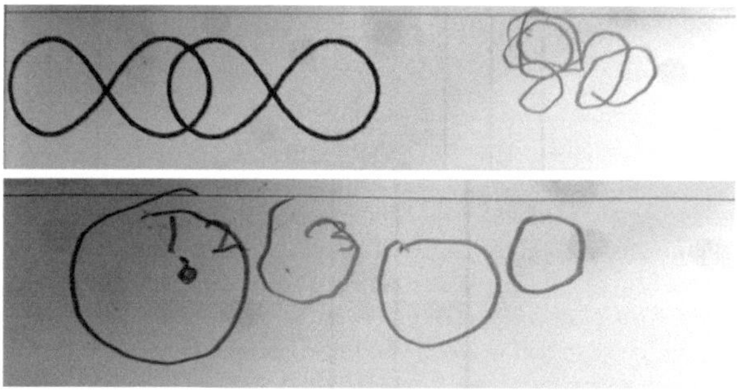

Fig. 4.3 Examples of constructional dyspraxia (copy infinity diagram, clock drawing)

more prominent features. This pattern of visuospatial impairment is most consistent with posterior cortical involvement. AB's language performance, with relatively better object and picture naming ability, and impaired comprehension are also suggestive of involvement of posterior cortical regions underpinning language, namely, the angular gyrus. See Table 4.1.

When considered together with concordant findings in structural as well as functional neuroimaging, a diagnosis of posterior cortical atrophy (PCA) was considered most appropriate. Dementia with Lewy bodies (DLB) was thought to be less likely given the lack of fluctuation over time and the absence of visual hallucinations. The absence of parkinsonian signs and symptoms made the diagnosis of corticobasal degeneration (CBD) unlikely as well, and the paucity of cerebrovascular changes on brain MRI made diminished the likelihood of vascular etiology in this case.

Discussion

PCA as a clinical syndrome was first described in a series of five cases wherein the presentation was characterized by relatively restricted, progressive deficits in higher-order visual processing with evidence of parieto-occipital atrophy on brain imaging [4]. Notably, episodic memory, verbal fluency and insight, and linguistic ability remain reasonably well preserved in early stages of the disease, setting the syndrome of PCA apart from more "typical" amnestic variants of the Alzheimer's disease phenotype. In considering the underlying neuropathological process, one of the largest series reporting pathological data on 21 patients found that 16 of these patients had underlying Alzheimer's disease. The 16 cases included 5 in which there was mixed AD/DLB/Parkinson's disease pathology. Diagnoses in the remaining five cases were prion disease (2), CBD (2), and subcortical gliosis (1) [5]. PCA in the majority of cases can therefore be viewed as lying on a phenotypic continuum of other AD phenotypes. Other PCA neuropathological subtypes in this series included CBD, DLB, and prion disease.

PCA is characterized by prominent decline in visuospatial and visual perceptual functions, alexia, and features of Balint's (simultanagnosia, ocular apraxia,

Table 4.1 Diagnostic criteria for posterior cortical atrophy

Core features	Supportive features
1. Insidious onset and gradual progression of cognitive deficits 2. The patient typically presents with visual complaints and shows evidence of disabling visual impairment in the absence of ocular disease 3. Episodic memory, verbal fluency, and insight are relatively preserved in the early stages of the disorder 4. One or more of the following features are present: (a) Simultanagnosia with or without optic ataxia or ocular apraxia (b) Constructional dyspraxia (c) Visual field defect (d) Environmental disorientation (e) Features of Gerstmann's syndrome (dysgraphia, dyscalculia, finger agnosia, right-left disorientation) 5. Absence of early parkinsonism or hallucinations 6. Absence of stroke or tumor	1. Alexia 2. Ideomotor or dressing apraxia 3. Prosopagnosia 4. Onset before age 65 years 5. Neuroimaging evidence: (a) Focal or asymmetric atrophy in the parietal and/or occipital regions (b) Focal or asymmetric hypoperfusion/hypometabolism in the parietal and/or occipital regions

Adapted from Mendez et al. [2] and Tang-Wai et al. [3]

optic ataxia, environmental agnosia) and Gerstmann's (left-right disorientation, agraphia, acalculia, and finger agnosia) syndromes [6]. The clinical presentation often reflects this underlying pattern of neuropsychological dysfunction, as in the case of our patient. An early history of visual symptoms is likely to be obtained, with patients reporting problems with reading, judging distances (leading at times to motor vehicle accidents), or having difficulty negotiating stairs or escalators. Patients may also report declining ability to use common objects suggestive of dyspraxia. With disease progression and when cortical atrophy becomes more widespread, frontal, executive, and memory impairments become apparent. AB had been noted to decline over a few years, and this relatively long history would likely account for his more widespread impairment revealed on neuropsychological assessment.

PCA is an uncommon debilitating focal neurodegenerative syndrome, associated most commonly with AD neuropathology, though also attributable to CBD, DLB, or prion disease [5]. Patients can often present to the ophthalmologist given the prominence of visual symptoms, and misdiagnosis can lead to wrong interventions being offered. Given the relative preservation of insight and memory, patients can benefit greatly from appropriate referral to occupational therapists, who can assist with compensatory strategies similar to those applied in persons with partial sightedness or blindness. Group and individual psychological approaches as well as psychoeducation for the patient and their families are of importance as well. There is a lack of systematic evidence for the use of pharmacological strategies such as cholinesterase inhibitors in delaying the progression of cognitive deficits, though comorbid anxiety or depression would need to be recognized and treated appropriately.

Acknowledgments The authors thank Sophia Dean for helping with manuscript preparation.

References

1. Addenbrooke's Cognitive Examination. ACE III Australian Version A. 2012 (updated 2012 Nov 11). Available at: http://neura.edu.au/sites/neura.edu.au/files/page-downloads/ACE-III%20Administration%20(Australian).pdf.
2. Mendez MF, Ghajarania M, Perryman KM. Posterior cortical atrophy: clinical characteristics and differences compared to Alzheimer's disease. Dement Geriatr Cogn Disord. 2002;14(1):33–40.
3. Tang-Wai DF, Graff-Radford NR, Boeve BF, Dickson DW, Parisi JE, Crook R, Caselli RJ, Knopman DS, Petersen RC. Clinical, genetic, and neuropathologic characteristics of posterior cortical atrophy. Neurology. 2004;63(7):1168–74.
4. Benson DF, Davis RJ, Snyder BD. Posterior cortical atrophy. Arch Neurol. 1988;45(7): 789–93.
5. Renner JA, Burns JM, Hou CE, McKeel DW, Storandt M, Morris JC. Progressive posterior cortical dysfunction a clinicopathologic series. Neurology. 2004;63(7):1175–80.
6. Crutch SJ, Lehmann M, Schott JM, Rabinovici GD, Rossor MN, Fox NC. Posterior cortical atrophy. Lancet Neurol. 2012;11(2):170–8.

Chapter 5
Posterior Cortical Atrophy (PCA)

Tillmann Supprian

At the age of 49 years, Mrs. A. first realized significant impairment in common daily activities. While renovating a room in her house, she was not able to adequately measure the length of a carpet. She couldn't handle the folding rule correctly and was not able to read the actual length. She could not explain the failure and was ashamed.

Being a mother of three and working part-time as a clerk, "burnout" was assumed, and she was hospitalized for a couple of weeks in a psychosomatic clinic. However, handicaps were progressive: at instances, she couldn't read the clock. She wasn't able to tie her shoes anymore and occasionally struggled when dressing. After washing clothes, she had problems to untangle twisted sleeves. At work, she had trouble when dialing phone numbers: she was switching numbers and had to concentrate hard to avoid mistakes. She stopped driving after she failed to back out from her garage. At the age of 52, she fell upon her face and broke her nose while walking with her dog. The accident happened because she stumbled across the dog. She also reported to feel insecure when walking. A CT scan was performed with no remarkable results.

Background History

Family history was empty for dementia. Her mother was nearly 80 years old and healthy; her father had died at an age of 72 because of a sepsis. A brother had died in his 40s from myocardial infarction. Her infancy and childhood were normal; she suffered no severe diseases during her life. Her intellectual development was reported to be unremarkable; she was sent to school regularly at the age of 7, finished high school, and then performed an education as civil servant at the tax office.

T. Supprian, MD, PhD
Section of Geriatric Psychiatry, Department of Psychiatry and Psychotherapy, Medical Faculty, Heinrich-Heine University, Düsseldorf, Germany
e-mail: Tillmann.Supprian@lvr.de

J. Priller, H. Rickards (eds.), *Neuropsychiatry Case Studies*,
DOI 10.1007/978-3-319-42190-2_5

Examination

She was fully alert, oriented, and in sub-depressed mood. Her report was structured and thinking was logical. She showed no tendencies of exaggeration or simulation. Concentration was good and stable over time. Short-term and long-term memory was normal. Language was fluent although she complained of occasional difficulties finding words. Reading was very slowly, and she made a couple of mistakes in the pronunciation of difficult words. Calculation was not significantly impaired. Sleep was reported to be normal. She never experienced hallucinations. With regard to current political and social events, her knowledge was relatively poor, and she explained that she was not interested in news, neither from newspapers nor from TV.

Initial Investigations

At her first consultation of a neurologist, an EEG showed ß-activity and was interpreted as a normal variant. Because of her depressed mood, self-doubt, lack of initiative, and thrive, a SSRI was prescribed, but had little effect. During the follow-up over 1 year, the neurologist became convinced that her complaints were due to an organic brain disease and not "psychogenic."

Progress

Neuropsychological testing was performed at the age of 53 together with cerebral MRI and CSF. Her premorbid verbal intelligence was tested with the MWT-B ("Mehrfachwahl-Wortschatz-Test", a German instrument for the assessment of verbal intelligence), and she scored above average. The mini-mental status test score was 25 and was suspicious with regard to her age. The clock-drawing test was severely impaired and indicated "dementia." However, results of the DemTect (a German neuropsychological screening instrument using verbal learning tasks, verbal fluency, and other cognitive domains) showed normal cognitive functions. Also the results of the Wechsler Memory Test (WMT), which is very sensitive for Alzheimer's dementia, were normal.

CSF showed elevated tau protein and reduced ß-amyloid, thus a typical finding of Alzheimer's disease. The MRI scan report described mild general brain atrophy, but no hippocampal atrophy, no vascular or inflammatory lesions, and no malformation. The MRI scan is given in Fig. 5.1.

Differential Diagnosis

Ophthalmological assessment was performed several times after the onset of her visual complaints with no pathological findings except myopia. Her glasses were changed, but this had no effect on her vision. A visual field defect was excluded by perimetry.

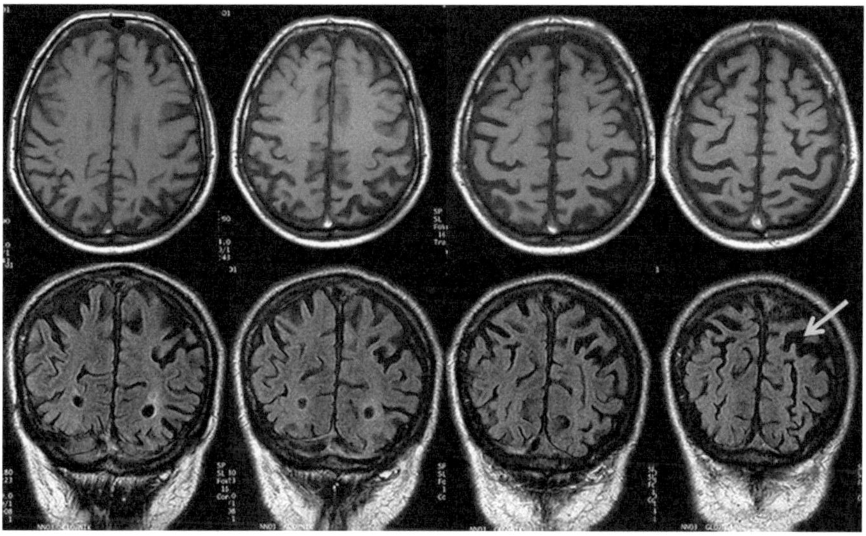

Fig. 5.1 T1-weighted MRI scan (*upper line* axial angulation, *left* is caudal, *right* is dorsal; *lower line* coronal angulation, *left* is rostral, *right* is occipital). Note the widening of sulci, especially on the right side (*white arrow*) (MRI scan with friendly permission from Prof. Dr. C. Will, Bocholt)

Further Investigation

In addition to the MRI, the neurologist initiated a FDG-PET, which was performed at an external institution (see Fig. 5.2).

This PET scan was reported to show typical parieto-occipital hypometabolism of Alzheimer's disease. No comment was made on the right/left difference of parietal metabolism. Together with the CSF findings and the heterogenous neuropsychological test results, early-onset Alzheimer's disease was diagnosed. The diagnosis was discussed by the neurologist with the patient and her spouse. The confirmatory PET scan result depressed the patient very much, since she doubted the diagnosis of Alzheimer's disease from the beginning. She had informed herself on Alzheimer's disease and realized many differences to her own impairments. Totally aware of her visual complaints, she had no memory loss.

Because she and her husband questioned the diagnosis of Alzheimer's disease and neuropsychological tests did indeed show contradictory results, the neurologist referred her to our memory clinic for further evaluation.

Diagnosis

Insidious onset and slow progression of symptoms indicated a neurodegenerative disorder. We ordered copies of the MRI scan for reevaluation by our neuroradiologist. Circumscribed brain atrophy of parieto-occipital gyri, especially in the right

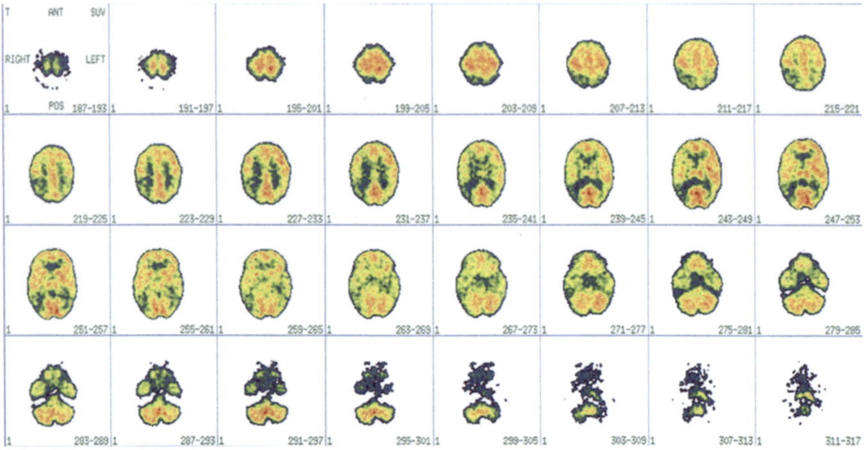

Fig. 5.2 Axial FDG-PET scan. Note the asymmetry in uptake, with hypometabolism in the right parietal region (*black arrow*) (PET scan with friendly permission from Dr. C. Naegele, Oberhausen)

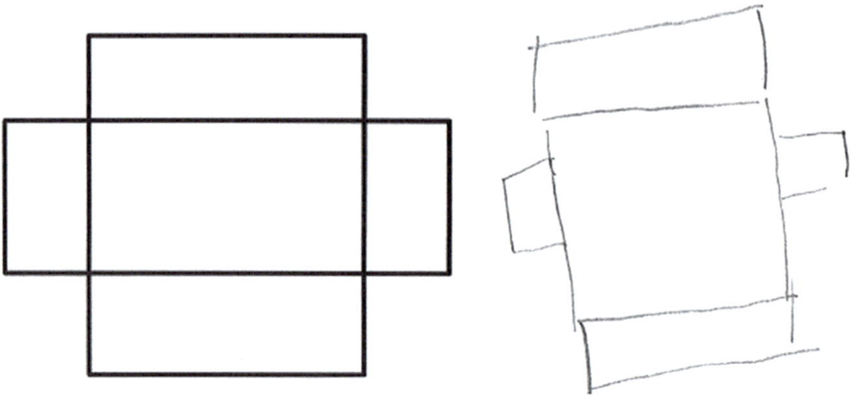

Fig. 5.3 Copying figures: original pattern on the *left*, copy of patient on the *right*

hemisphere, corresponded to asymmetry of metabolism on the PET scan. Thus, a focal parieto-occipital brain atrophy typical for posterior cortical atrophy (PCA) was diagnosed.

Clinical presentation indicated impairments especially in visuospatial and visuoperceptual domains. When presented with complex visual material, she was significantly handicapped. She couldn't follow even very simple comic strips. Thus, she identified some isolated objects on the pictures, but was not able to comprehend the complete scene. Among the neuropsychological tests, the most severe impairment was found when she was asked to copy figures (Fig. 5.3).

What Did I Learn from This Case?

I learned that the diagnosis of early-onset Alzheimer's disease was a severe distress for Mrs. A. because she had certain beliefs regarding this disorder, which frightened her very much. When the diagnosis was specified to PCA, she better understood her impairments and could comprehend the differences to typical Alzheimer's dementia. However, she still had many questions regarding the origin of this rare disorder and the prognosis. She asked for literature, and it was hard to find nonscientific German literature suitable for a patient. We did not recommend her to join an Alzheimer support group, because her disorder differed so much from typical AD patients. The patient and her spouse were very much interested in therapeutic concepts such as neuropsychological training to compensate her impairments.

I also learned that brain imaging is pivotal in the diagnostic process of neurodegenerative disorders and interpretation of MRI scans in rare disorders such as PCA requires a lot of experience. The initial written report of the MRI scan didn't describe the focal atrophy of parieto-occipital gyri, and the PET scan report didn't mention asymmetry in metabolism. It is important to discuss images between clinicians and neuroradiologists.

Finally, I've learned that visual problems without ocular abnormalities require extensive neurological evaluation.

Bibliography

Borruat FX. Posterior cortical atrophy: review of the recent literature. Curr Neurol Neurosci Rep. 2013;13:406.

Crutch SJ, Lehmann M, Schott JM, Rabinovici GD, Rossor MN, Fox NC. Posterior cortical atrophy. Lancet Neurol. 2012;11:170–8.

Goldstein MA, Ivanov I, Silverman ME. Posterior cortical atrophy: an exemplar for renovating diagnostic formulation in neuropsychiatry. Compr Psychiatry. 2011;52:326–33.

Chapter 6
Case Study: Little Red Riding Hood

Marlies Baldee-Hordijk and Erik van Duijn

Introduction

Mrs. B, 68 years old, was referred by her general practitioner (GP) since she had sudden attacks of laughing and shaking, mostly occurring after lunch. The GP described her mental condition as "hysterical," but he was also concerned about her physical condition. Her GP suspected a malignancy because she had lost weight and was looking unhealthy. Since she was a heavy smoker, the GP suspected a lung malignancy with possible metastases and requested imaging of her lungs, as the patient had refused this so far.

History

Mrs. B. had a troubled youth, and she got married against her will at the age of 18. She had three children and still lived with her husband despite of continuous relationship problems. She had worked as a mental health nurse until her first hospitalization on a psychiatric ward at the age of 30. In the past four decades, she had been diagnosed with borderline personality disorder, dysthymic disorder, dissociative disorder, relationship problems, as well as alcohol and benzodiazepine dependence. She also had physical problems and was diagnosed with hypothyroidism, fibromyalgia, and osteoarthritis. Her last hospitalization was at the age of 61, and until then she had been hospitalized 29 times, most of the time because of increased suicidality or alcohol abuse. During the last 7 years, her mental condition was relatively stable, and she received outpatient care for symptoms and behavior that were associated with her borderline personality disorder. A psychiatric nurse visited her at home monthly.

M. Baldee-Hordijk, MD
Centre for Mental Health Care Delfland, Delft, The Netherlands
e-mail: m.baldee-hordijk@ggz-delfland.nl

E. van Duijn, MD, PhD (✉)
Centre for Mental Health Care Delfland, Leiden University Medical Centre, Delft, The Netherlands
e-mail: e.vanduijn@ggz-delfland.nl

J. Priller, H. Rickards (eds.), *Neuropsychiatry Case Studies*,
DOI 10.1007/978-3-319-42190-2_6

Examination

During one of the home visits, Mrs. B. suddenly started laughing at the nurse and the psychiatrist for no apparent reason. She giggled to the nurse who was wearing a red blouse and to the psychiatrist: "There you have Little Red Riding Hood and the Wolf!" She showed childish euphoria and excitement. After a mental examination, the patient said that nothing was wrong with her and she was feeling well. She emphasized that she had no physical complaints. Yet, her husband and daughter expressed their worries and described that she had almost every day periods of laughter and crying since 2 months and that she was experiencing attacks of uncontrollable shaking several times a day. She went compulsively to the bathroom without any reason. She drank up to 1.5 l of soft drinks (coke) per day, and despite this, she had lost 5 kg (almost 10 %) of weight. She had decreased self-care and hygiene. During the mental examination, she was uncooperative, and she was laughing almost continuously, for which she apologized but failed to stop doing so. She made inappropriate (sexual) comments toward the psychiatrist and the nurse. She had a good orientation and her memory had no large gaps. She showed increased distraction, whereas her perception was undisturbed and her thinking was coherent. Her mood seemed to be normal without symptoms of (hypo)mania, but she showed a marked inappropriate affect. She expressed moderate insight in her uncommon behavior. Neurological examination was normal.

Initial Investigations

Routine blood screening showed a slightly lowered folic acid 4.7 nmol/l (normal >5.0 nmol/l) and a vitamin D deficiency 24 nmol/l (normal 50–185 nmol/l), but no further abnormalities. The mini-mental state examination (MMSE) score was 29 out of 30. The Frontal Assessment Battery (FAB) scored 9 out of 18. During the verbal fluency test, she said only five (Dutch) words with the letter "S," all with a strong provocative meaning like "sucker." She drew a small clock of only 3.5 cm (Fig. 6.1, clock 1) and refused to draw a larger one. She drew the numbers up to nine and then realized that she had no space left for the remaining numbers. The hands of the clock were drawn incorrectly as shown in Fig. 6.1.

Differential Diagnosis

Since she showed noticeable disinhibited and social inappropriate behavior and decreased self-care, and she had a low score on the FAB, with an almost perfect MMSE score, the differential diagnosis included frontal cerebral pathology such as frontotemporal dementia or brain malignancy. Although she did not show evident mood changes, a bipolar disorder was part of the differential diagnosis because of the periods of uncontrollable laughing and euphoria, associative expression about Little Red Riding Hood, and her uninhibited, provocative verbal responses during the tests.

Fig. 6.1 Subject's first drawing of a clock

Also, it could not be excluded that her behavioral changes were unusual symptoms of her borderline personality disorder at that time. Furthermore, the sudden attacks of shaking could be symptoms of epileptic convulsions or a conversion disorder.

Progress

The CT scan of the cerebrum showed no brain malignancy but widespread frontal atrophy that indicated frontotemporal dementia (Fig. 6.2). The X-ray of the lungs showed no abnormalities. Unfortunately, the patient refused further neuropsychological assessment, MRI, or EEG at that moment. Only after 2 years, she agreed to do additional investigations when she was seen by a neurologist again because of an increase of the shaking.

Further Investigation

The MRI cerebrum showed a slightly widened ventricular system, a global atrophy stage 2/3, mesiotemporal atrophy stage 2, and parietal atrophy stage 2 (Fig. 6.3a, b). There were almost no white matter lesions, no recent ischemia, and no signs of bleeding. The EEG showed a slightly slow/delayed background pattern with diffuse slow activity. The neuropsychological assessment showed mainly a dysfunction in executive cognitive function with visuoconstructive impairments and a limitation in language comprehension. She also had slight memory problems. A second clock-drawing test showed a similar outcome as 2 years earlier (Fig. 6.4, clock 2).

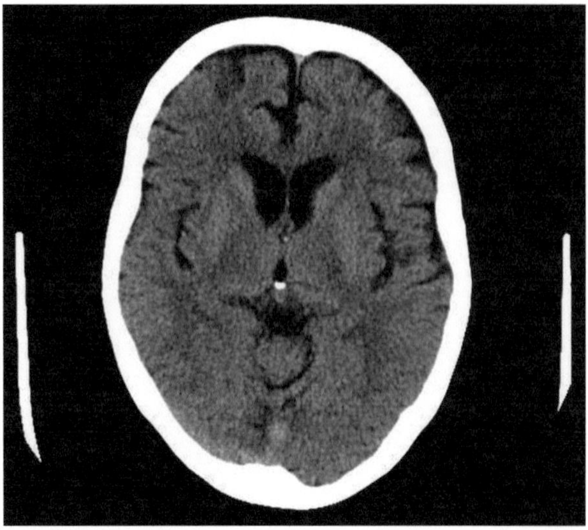

Fig. 6.2 The CT scan of the cerebrum showed no brain malignancy but widespread frontal atrophy that indicated frontotemporal dementia

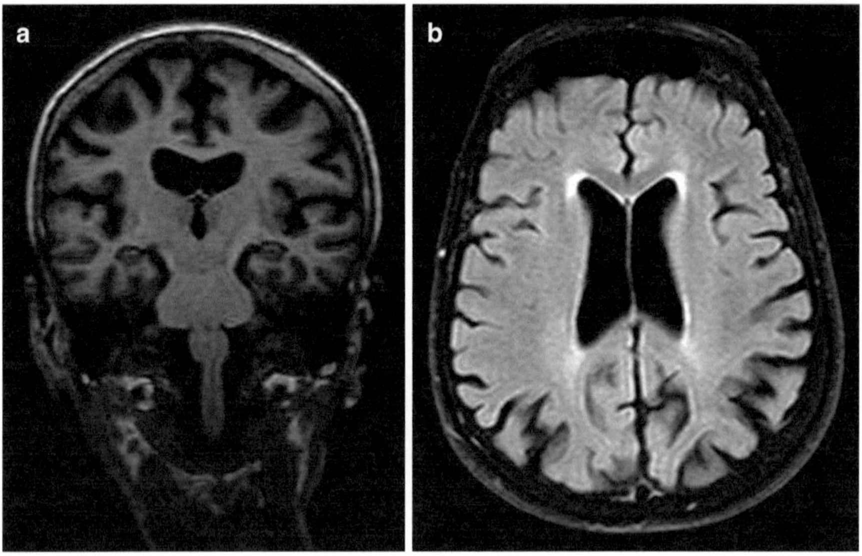

Fig. 6.3 (**a**, **b**) The MRI cerebrum showed a slightly widened ventricular system, a global atrophy stage 2/3, mesiotemporal atrophy stage 2, and parietal atrophy stage 2

Diagnosis

Given the progressive behavioral changes and the results of imaging and neuropsychological assessments, she was diagnosed with the behavioral variant of frontotemporal dementia. No explanation was found for the shaking attacks.

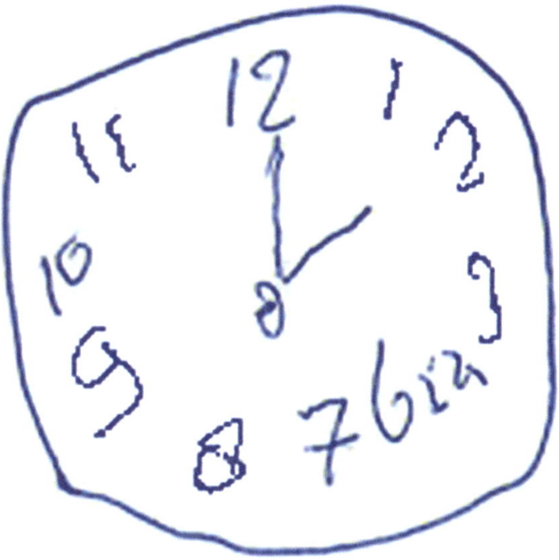

Fig. 6.4 Subject's second drawing of a clock

What Did I Learn from This Case?

If a patient with a chronic psychiatric disorder shows new atypical behavior, it is important to consider neurological causes of the changed clinical presentation. A literature search resulted in a case report that described "moria" (foolish or silly euphoria) and "Witzelsucht" (tendency to tell inappropriate jokes) in a person with frontotemporal dementia [1], a condition that was similar to the laughing and euphoria in our patient. Since it may be difficult to differentiate early manifestations of frontotemporal dementia from other psychiatric disorders with prominent behavioral problems, including borderline personality disorders and mood disorders, assessment of cognitive functioning should be considered. When a patient is not able or willing to do a comprehensive neuropsychological test, the clock-drawing test or the FAB is useful as screening instruments.

Reference

1. Mendez MF. Moria and Witzelsucht from frontotemporal dementia. J Neuropsychiatr Clin Neurosci. 2005;17:429–30.

Chapter 7
Not All Unusual Behavior Is Psychotic

Kevin Foy

BD was a 53-year-old man referred for a neuropsychiatric opinion after being admitted to a general psychiatric ward on section. The referral stated that he was depressed, was not speaking, and was adopting unusual postures and hadn't responded to previous antidepressant or antipsychotic medications.

Background

From reviewing his notes, it was clear that he had no previous psychiatric history until a year earlier. He had worked as a librarian and had been sacked some months previously after unusual behavior at work. The behavior included photocopying large NASA reports, damaging a photocopier when paper jammed, taking extra breaks at work, and hiding in the office.

His general practitioner referred him to mental health services with a history of anxiety and depression after he had lost his job. At initial psychiatry assessment, he appeared quite preoccupied with themes of science fiction. At that assessment, it was noted that his speech was disjointed and difficult to follow. He denied any anxiety or depression. The psychiatrist felt that he had a psychotic illness with thought disorder and started him on an antidepressant and antipsychotic medication.

Over a period of 6 months, further follow-up appointments revealed that his partner expressed some concerns relating to his memory, as well as his motivation and interaction with others. She also felt that there was a change in his personality, and he was increasingly isolated and quiet.

He was eventually sectioned under the mental health act due to increasing levels of apathy, reduced drive, and increased drinking of alcohol. By this stage, he was prescribed risperidone 6 mg once daily. He was eating limited amounts of food and was consuming more alcohol. The medical notes also mentioned that he was doubly incontinent and was neglecting his self-care. He was observed to be restless. He was also presenting with a continued grimace/twitch on his face and was believed to be unable to keep his jaw still.

K. Foy, MB, BCh, BAO, MSc, MRCPI, MRCPsych
The Walton Centre NHS Foundation Trust, Liverpool, UK
e-mail: kevin.foy@thewaltoncentre.nhs.uk

J. Priller, H. Rickards (eds.), *Neuropsychiatry Case Studies*,
DOI 10.1007/978-3-319-42190-2_7

Since Admission

The inpatient team found it difficult to communicate with him. He had been started on a new antipsychotic medication with no real improvement.

At Time of Assessment

A collateral history from nurses reported that he was extremely apathetic all of the time. He required high levels of prompting, and even with prompting, he didn't complete his care needs. He spent a lot of the time on his own and didn't socialize with anyone on the ward. He was intermittently incontinent of both urine and also feces. The staff encouraged him to eat by leaving a pack of sandwiches on his bed which he would consume in his own time. There was no evidence of depression or psychosis. He initially had a problem of grimacing, but this settled after his risperidone was reduced. There was no posturing, negativism, echolalia, echopraxia, etc. There was no deterioration or improvement in his symptoms since admission.

Mental State Examination

On mental state examination, he came across as a middle-aged man with a beard and long dirty finger nails. He was lying in bed with the curtains closed around him. He had limited interactions and no spontaneous speech. He was mildly perseverative in some hand gestures and also in saying no. He was oriented in time and place. He was able to say the day, month, and year all correctly and was just 1 day out on date. He said he didn't know the reason why he was in hospital but wasn't distressed at being there. He denied problems with his memory. He denied any low mood or psychotic phenomena. He denied any physical problems. He denied any headaches, weakness, respiratory, or GI problems. He was markedly apathetic and disinterested in the presence of others.

Cognitive Assessment

On cognitive assessment, he was slow at registering five words. Delayed word recall was zero out of five. He was able to name simple common objects, but naming for complex objects was poor. On semantic fluency, he was unable to list any words beginning with the letter F. On categorical fluency, he was unable to list any animals. Due to the challenges in interacting with him, testing of visuospatial functions and semantic memory wasn't possible. See Fig. 7.1.

The CT brain scan performed over 6 months ago and initially reported as "showing widespread ischemia" showed severe and dramatic frontal atrophy with some

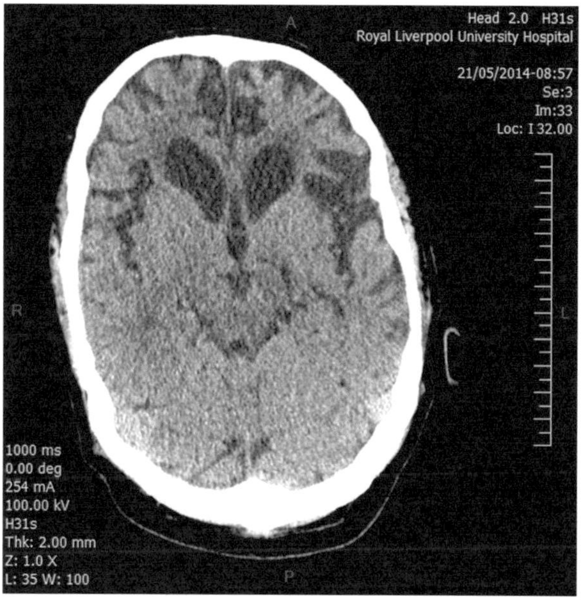

Fig. 7.1 Severe frontal lobe atrophy

hydrocephalus ex-vacuo of the frontal horns of the lateral ventricle and to a lesser extent some temporal lobe atrophy.

Diagnosis

Mr. BD was a 53-year-old man with at least a 2-year history of progressive deterioration in his functioning with personality change and increasing levels of apathy and decline in self-care with resultant high levels of self-neglect. He wasn't depressed, and his mood was on the whole very flat with no spontaneity or interest in interactions with other people or his environment. On assessment, he was oriented in time or place. His CT scan done over 6 months ago showed dramatic and very severe atrophy which was limited mainly to the frontal and a lesser extent temporal lobe. His presentation was that of a behavioral variant type of frontotemporal dementia. See Table 7.1.

What Did I Learn from This Case?

I noted the importance of being rather skeptical about the contents of referral notes as this referral note looked more like that of someone with catatonia than frontotemporal dementia. This case emphasized the importance of reviewing in detail the history and getting collateral information. Many CT scans are reviewed by

Table 7.1 Red flags for frontotemporal dementia

Personality changes
Increasing apathy and disinterest in activities
New onset impulsivity and risk-taking behavior
Changes in sense of humor with increased jocularity or immature behavior
Loss of empathy and social behavior
Cognitive deficits
Loss or changes in the ability to work or hold down a job
Reduced ability to organize their lives or manage things at home
Increasing forgetfulness
Communication problems – increasing difficulties in word-finding abilities or expressing themselves verbally
Physical signs
Urinary incontinence
Changes in gait
Presence of primitive reflexes, for example, grasp reflex

radiologists with limited neuroradiological training, and this case shows the importance of reviewing scans in a multidisciplinary way between the radiologist and the clinician.

Bibliography

Karageorgiou E, Miller BL. Frontotemporal lobar degeneration: a clinical approach. Semin Neurol. 2014;34(2):189–201. doi:10.1055/s-0034-1381735.

Kirshner HS. Frontotemporal dementia and primary progressive aphasia, a review. Neuropsychiatr Dis Treat. 2014;10:1045–55. doi:10.2147/NDT.S38821.

Pressman PS, Miller BL. Diagnosis and management of behavioral variant frontotemporal dementia. Biol Psychiatry. 2014;75(7):574–81. doi:10.1016/j.biopsych.2013.11.006.

Chapter 8
Puzzling Case: Is the Answer in the Genes?

Emma Devenney and John Hodges

Case Vignette

A 54-year-old male retired public servant was referred to the frontotemporal dementia clinic in 2008 with a history of insidious change in personality and behavior spanning over a decade. His wife first noticed a change in his personality in the late 1990s. He began to overspend on unnecessary items, and they lost their house when he failed to pay the mortgage. Over the ensuing few years, he was imprisoned on three occasions for fraudulent behavior. He was disinhibited in social situations, at times in a sexual manner. He held grandiose delusions about himself, for example, he often described himself as a champion bowler. On one occasion, he reported that he had been abducted in a helicopter and drugged which is why he had not appeared in court. In contrast to relatively preserved motivation, his ability to empathize and sympathize was profoundly reduced. He preferred to spend time alone. He could be mentally rigid, secretive, and at times aggressive.

The patient had no insight into these problems. Instead, he complained of recent difficulties with balance and mild long-standing memory complaints since a motorcycle accident in 1982. He was moderately impaired for activities of daily living (ADLs).

E. Devenney, MB, BCh, BAO, MRCP • J. Hodges, MBBS, FRCPF, MedSci, FRACP (✉)
Neuroscience Research Australia, Sydney, NSW, Australia
e-mail: e.devenney@neura.edu.au; j.hodges@neura.edu.au

J. Priller, H. Rickards (eds.), *Neuropsychiatry Case Studies*,
DOI 10.1007/978-3-319-42190-2_8

Background

Medical History

His past medical history was significant for a head and neck injury following the motorcycle accident 30 years previously. He required ongoing treatment with opiates to control neck pain and sensory disturbances in the right arm. He was unable to return to work following this.

Social History

He had a high-functioning job in the public sector until his accident meant he could no longer work. According to his wife, during the early years of marriage, he was astute with finances, had no trouble with the law, and showed no signs of disinhibition. Their marriage was happy; they had an active social life, enjoyed sporting activities, and had many friends.

Family History

His mother was diagnosed with parkinsonism in late life that may have been accompanied by cognitive decline. His father may have had a psychotic episode that was attributed to a "ministroke." During this episode, his father reported seeing a man watching him from across the street when there was no one there. There is no other family history of neurodegenerative disorders.

Examination

On physical examination, there was evidence of mild symmetrical parkinsonism with rigidity and bradykinesia, but without tremor. There were no ALS features or evidence of apraxia.

General cognitive screening tests revealed overall mild impairment (Addenbrooke's Cognitive Examination – 79/100). On more formal cognitive tests, he showed severe impairments in learning and memory, confrontation naming, and visuoconstruction and on measures of executive function (including verbal fluency and switching between two trains of thought). Borderline impairment was also noted in working memory, in verbal comprehension, and on an executive measure of inhibitory control. By contrast, his attentional, language reception, word repetition, and basic visuoperceptual skills remained within normal limits. On a self-report measure of mood, he reported normal (i.e., low) levels of depression, anxiety, and stress symptoms.

Investigations

A structural MRI of the brain did not reveal any evidence of significant focal atrophy (Fig. 8.1). A subsequent FDG-PET revealed equivocal reduced uptake in the medial frontal lobes.

Differential Diagnosis

The behavioral features in this case were suggestive of behavioral variant frontotemporal dementia (bvFTD), but there were a number of unusual features. Firstly, the clinical course was protracted and indolent spanning over 20 years. In addition, the lack of significant frontal or temporal changes on either structural or metabolic imaging was completely at odds with a diagnosis of bvFTD [1]. According to international diagnostic criteria for bvFTD, imaging changes are necessary for progression from possible to probable bvFTD [2].

There is no doubt that he had cognitive deficits on testing, but there were a number of other possible etiologies for this including the effects of his prior head and neck injury and long-standing opiate usage.

There are a subgroup of men who have symptoms of FTD but show no brain atrophy and no progression over many years known as “phenocopy” cases. The etiology in these cases is uncertain, but a proportion has long-standing personality disorders which decompensate in midlife. In keeping with a diagnosis of “phenocopy syndrome,” this case lacked definite abnormalities on MRI and PET [3]. Unlike typical phenocopy cases, however, this patient did show impairment on

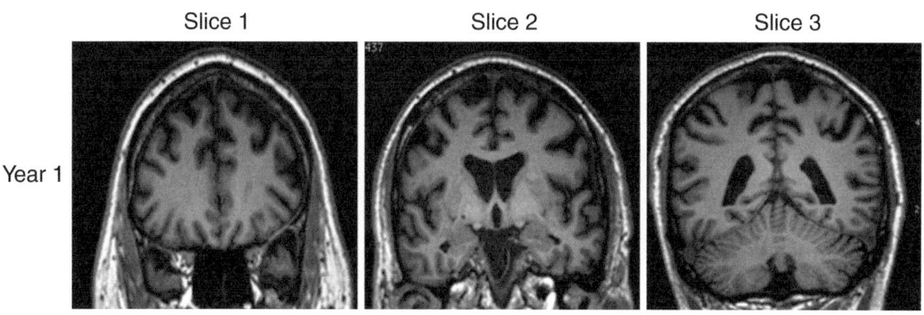

Fig. 8.1 Coronal T1 images at the orbitofrontal cortex (slice 1), the anterior temporal lobe (slice 2), and precuneus and cerebellum (slice 3) at presentation (year 1)

general and more specific cognitive tasks which have shown good sensitivity to true bvFTD [4, 5]. His ADLs were moderately impaired which is also against the "phenocopy syndrome" diagnosis [6].

Follow-Up

He was reviewed on an annual basis for the subsequent 4 years and during this time after he remained disinhibited with increasingly sexualized behaviors. He continued to overspend, and his stories became increasingly delusional. He became apathetic, exhibited obvious memory problems, and was disoriented at most recent review.

Further Investigations

There was little progression on MRI until 2012. At this time, atrophy was unequivocally present and involved the frontal and parietal regions (Fig. 8.2).

Genetic testing in 2012 for the newly discovered C9orf72 genetic mutation was positive.

Diagnosis

The diagnosis of bvFTD associated with the C9orf72 mutation was made based on the progressive clinical and MRI changes and genetic testing. The discovery of this new genetic mutation in bvFTD has facilitated a definitive diagnosis in a number of diagnostically challenging cases, and a clinical phenotype for this mutation is beginning to emerge.

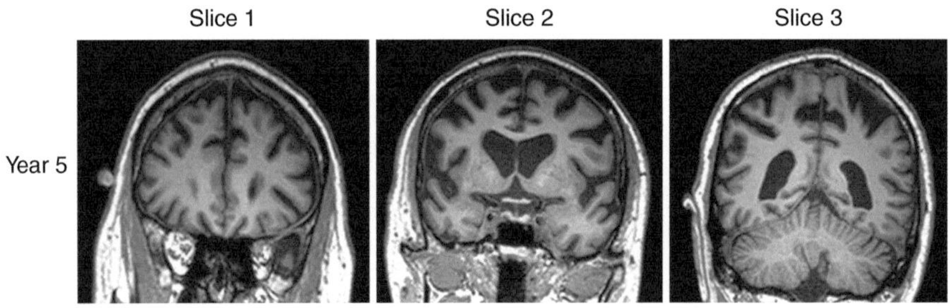

Fig. 8.2 Coronal T1 images at the orbitofrontal cortex (slice 1), the anterior temporal lobe (slice 2), and precuneus and cerebellum (slice 3) at follow-up (year 5)

Learning Points

This case highlighted important considerations to be aware of when considering FTD in the context of the C9orf72 mutation and reminds us that not all cases fit neatly into one diagnostic category (Table 8.1).

A protracted clinical course was previously rarely encountered in cases of bvFTD, but we now know that survival rates in *C9orf72* can be variable, and survival up to 17 years has been reported [7]. The majority of FTD carriers conform to the behavioral variant of FTD (bvFTD) although progressive nonfluent aphasia (PPA-nf) cases have also been noted. As in this case, the presence of prominent psychotic features appears to be a hallmark of this syndrome [8, 9] and can lead to a misdiagnosis of late-onset psychiatric disease. The family history also provides an important clue to the presence of this mutation. While not all families have a history of FTD, at least one half of bvFTD mutation-positive patients described a family history of ALS [9, 10], as well as a number of carriers describing significant psychiatric illness in family members [9].

While some genetic mutations are associated with distinct neuroimaging signatures, cortical gray matter changes in *C9orf72* mutation carriers appear to be heterogeneous. Almost every study has described subcortical atrophy particularly

Table 8.1 Characteristics of the C9orf72 mutation

Age of onset (years)		45–65
Survival (years)		1–17
Phenotype	bvFTD	+++
	PNFA	+
	SD	±
	FTD-MND	+++
	MND	+++
Clinical features	Lack of insight	+++
	Disinhibition	+++
	Apathy	+++
	Loss of empathy/sympathy	+++
	Stereotyped behaviors	+++
	Change in dietary preferences	+++
	Psychosis	++
	Executive dysfunction	++
	Memory dysfunction	++
Imaging findings		Variable. Ranging from normal findings on MRI and metabolic imaging studies to atrophy and hypometabolism in frontal and temporal regions
Pathology		TDP-43 proteinopathy

involving the thalamus, but the pattern of cortical atrophy has been considerably more variable, ranging from frontal and temporal atrophy of typical bvFTD to non-existent atrophy at presentation [11, 12].

This case highlights the importance of long-term follow-up in diagnostically challenging cases. It could be argued that a definitive diagnosis in neurodegenerative conditions is purely academic as disease-modifying treatments are not yet available. A definitive diagnosis however can be extremely important as it allows appropriate access to services, benefits, and support networks for the patient and their families. In this case, the genetic information will allow subsequent generations to make informed life decisions.

References

1. Kipps CM, Hodges JR, Hornberger M. Nonprogressive behavioural frontotemporal dementia: recent developments and clinical implications of the 'bvFTD phenocopy syndrome'. Curr Opin Neurol. 2010;23(6):628–32.
2. Rascovsky K, Hodges JR, Kipps CM, Johnson JK, Seeley WW, Mendez MF, et al. Diagnostic criteria for the behavioral variant of frontotemporal dementia (bvFTD): current limitations and future directions. Alzheimer Dis Assoc Disord. 2007;21(4):S14–8.
3. Kipps CM, Hodges JR, Fryer TD, Nestor PJ. Combined magnetic resonance imaging and positron emission tomography brain imaging in behavioural variant frontotemporal degeneration: refining the clinical phenotype. Brain: J Neurol. 2009;132(Pt 9):2566–78.
4. Hornberger M, Piguet O, Kipps C, Hodges JR. Executive function in progressive and nonprogressive behavioral variant frontotemporal dementia. Neurology. 2008;71(19):1481–8.
5. Hornberger M, Shelley BP, Kipps CM, Piguet O, Hodges JR. Can progressive and non-progressive behavioural variant frontotemporal dementia be distinguished at presentation? J Neurol Neurosurg Psychiatry. 2009;80(6):591–3.
6. Mioshi E, Hsieh S, Savage S, Hornberger M, Hodges JR. Clinical staging and disease progression in frontotemporal dementia. Neurology. 2010;74(20):1591–7.
7. Irwin DJ, McMillan CT, Brettschneider J, Libon DJ, Powers J, Rascovsky K, et al. Cognitive decline and reduced survival in C9orf72 expansion frontotemporal degeneration and amyotrophic lateral sclerosis. J Neurol Neurosurg Psychiatry. 2013;84(2):163–9.
8. Snowden JS, Rollinson S, Thompson JC, Harris JM, Stopford CL, Richardson AM, et al. Distinct clinical and pathological characteristics of frontotemporal dementia associated with C9ORF72 mutations. Brain: J Neurol. 2012;135(Pt 3):693–708.
9. Devenney E, Hornberger M, Irish M, Mioshi E, Burrell J, Tan R, et al. Frontotemporal dementia associated with the C9ORF72 mutation: a unique clinical profile. JAMA Neurol. 2014;71(3):331–9.
10. Boeve BF, Boylan KB, Graff-Radford NR, DeJesus-Hernandez M, Knopman DS, Pedraza O, et al. Characterization of frontotemporal dementia and/or amyotrophic lateral sclerosis associated with the GGGGCC repeat expansion in C9ORF72. Brain: J Neurol. 2012;135(Pt 3):765–83.
11. Mahoney CJ, Beck J, Rohrer JD, Lashley T, Mok K, Shakespeare T, et al. Frontotemporal dementia with the C9ORF72 hexanucleotide repeat expansion: clinical, neuroanatomical and neuropathological features. Brain: J Neurol. 2012;135(Pt 3):736–50.
12. Irish M, Devenney E, Wong S, Dobson-Stone C, Kwok JB, Piguet O, et al. Neural substrates of episodic memory dysfunction in behavioural variant frontotemporal dementia with and without C9ORF72 expansions. Neuroimage Clin. 2013;2:836–43.

Part II
Movement Disorders

Chapter 9
Hallucinations in Parkinson's Disease

Roger A. Barker and Gemma Cummins

A 74-year-old male with a 7-year history of idiopathic Parkinson's disease presented with visual hallucinations and memory difficulties. One year ago, he started experiencing a "feeling of presence" of someone out of the corner of his eye. This sensation was fleeting and occurred once or twice per week. However, over recent months he was having more well-formed visual hallucinations, occurring on an almost daily basis. His wife had noted a significant deterioration in his memory over the last 2 years, whereby he was forgetting appointments and having difficulty in managing his medications and finances. He was becoming increasingly dependent on his family members for activities of daily living. He had a 10-year history of REM sleep behavior disturbance and tended to be sleepy during the day. His medications included co-benyldopa 25/100 qds, co-benyldopa-controlled release 25/100 OD nocte, and rasagiline 1 mg OD.

The patient described waking up at nighttime to go to the bathroom and seeing a group of men in suits and women in hats levitating over his bed. As he reached out to try and touch the images, they appeared to move further away from him. He also recounted an episode whereby it felt like he was walking through dense foliage in the corridor en route to the bathroom at night, and he felt he had to push tree branches aside to make his way through. On reaching the bathroom, he noted giant insects crawling out of the toilet bowl. At other times, he told his wife he could see purple cows in the garden when looking out the kitchen window. Usually the patient retained a degree of insight into these hallucinations and found them mildly amusing, but on occasion he reported the perceptual changes were more disturbing and frightened him, such as the time he saw a man hanging on his bedroom door at night. The hallucinations became more frequent and florid when he had been admitted to hospital 3 months previously for delirium secondary to a urinary tract infection. During this admission, he reported seeing multiple rows of eggs hatching small ducks that resembled the storybook character Jemima Puddle-Duck [1]. He denied any olfactory or auditory hallucinations or delusions and had no other psychiatric symptoms.

R.A. Barker, BA, MBBS, MRCP, PhD (✉) • G. Cummins, MB, MRCPI
John van Geest Centre for Brain Repair, Addenbrooke's Hospital, Cambridge, UK
e-mail: rab46@cam.ac.uk; gac54@cam.ac.uk

J. Priller, H. Rickards (eds.), *Neuropsychiatry Case Studies*,
DOI 10.1007/978-3-319-42190-2_9

On examination, the patient had typical parkinsonian features with hypomimia, cogwheel rigidity affecting both upper limbs, a resting tremor more pronounced in his right upper limb, and global bradykinesia. He walked with a stooped posture and mild festination. The pull test was normal with no signs of retropulsion. In addition to parkinsonism, the patient had marked cognitive problems. On neuropsychological examination, he was cooperative with preserved insight into his mental difficulties. Mini Mental State Examination (MMSE) score was 26/30. Addenbrooke's Cognitive Examination-Revised (ACE-R) score was 66/100 (attention and orientation 18/18, fluency 8/14, memory 18/26, language 13/26, visuospatial 9/16). He was unable to copy interlocking pentagons, and his ability to draw a clockface was impaired. His Beck Depression Inventory (BDI) revealed a score of 4, indicating no depression. He had attended the ophthalmologist recently who found no impairment of vision or pathological changes in either eye.

Treatment with the cholinesterase inhibitor rivastigmine was initiated at 1.5 mg BID and titrated up to 3 mg BID. Clonazepam was started at 0.5 mg OD for his REM sleep behavior disturbance. The patient's wife was advised to leave a light on in the corridor at night, as most of his hallucinations tended to occur after dark. Following this treatment at 6 months follow-up, his hallucinations had reduced significantly, and his wife reported no further enactment of dreams at night. His motor symptoms were stable. While his family felt he was less confused than previously, there was no detectable improvement in his performance on cognitive testing.

Discussion

This patient initially developed a movement disorder with slowing of gait, bradykinesia, asymmetrical rigidity, and tremor which was responsive to dopaminergic treatment. The REM sleep behavior disturbance that anteceded the patient developing classical motor features of PD is now well recognized as a premanifest or early feature of PD [2]. Based on the initial symptoms, a diagnosis of idiopathic Parkinson's disease was made. There were no atypical symptoms or features to suggest any other form of parkinsonism such as multiple systems atrophy, corticobasal degeneration, or progressive supranuclear palsy. Initial brain imaging did not show any ischemic lesions suggestive of vascular parkinsonism. He developed a gradual onset and successive worsening of cognitive impairment and hallucinations 5 years after initially manifesting parkinsonism. This was heralded by minor hallucinations ("a feeling of presence"), but these later evolved into complex visual hallucinations comprising of well-formed people and animals.

Dementia with Lewy bodies (DLB) can present with parkinsonism, dementia, and visual hallucinations, but the diagnostic criteria stipulate that cognitive impairment presents within 1 year of the onset of parkinsonism [3]. Patients with dementia beginning at least 1 year after the onset of motor symptoms are diagnosed with Parkinson's disease with dementia (PDD), and this is the most likely diagnosis in this patient. Pathologically, both DLB and PDD involve the accumulation of Lewy bodies in addition to cholinergic deficits, and many authors argue that the current clinical criteria used to discriminate between PDD and DLB are too arbitrary, as they are based mainly on the temporal relationship of the appearance of symptoms. It may be that both conditions represent different points on the continuum of "Lewy body disease" with a larger cortical burden of Lewy bodies in patients with DLB than PDD [4, 5].

PDD with Hallucinations

Hallucinations are a frequent neuropsychiatric symptom in PD with a high incidence and prevalence over time, affecting over 70 % of patients in a 20-year follow-up period [6]. They are more commonly found in alpha-synucleinopathies than the tauopathies or amyloidopathies [7]. They frequently herald progression to more severe forms of psychosis and dementia, with a 20-fold increase in the incidence of dementia over a 3-year period in PD patients with hallucinations compared to those without [8]. There is thus a well-established relationship between hallucinations and dementia in PD, and together they result in an increased need for nursing home placement and mortality [9]. The phenomenology of hallucinations changes through the course of the disease. In early PD, patients may experience minor hallucinations or delusions with well-preserved insight, but as the disease progresses, more structured, complex hallucinations predominate, and insight is often lost, particularly in patients with more severe cognitive impairment [10]. It is not unusual for patients to try to interact with the hallucinations. The visual hallucinations most often reported in PD consist of well-formed people, animals, or objects, with auditory, tactile, and olfactory hallucinations being comparatively rare [11].

Risk factors for developing hallucinations in PD are manifold and include older age, longer disease duration, greater severity of motor symptoms, depression, and other comorbidities [12]. In patients with PD and hallucinations, they very frequently have comorbid sleep disorders, including excessive daytime somnolence and REM sleep behavior disturbance. This had led to one hypothesis that the hallucinations could be caused by intrusions of REM sleep fragments into wakefulness and emergence of internally generated imagery [13, 14].

The pathophysiological mechanisms underlying hallucinations in PDD have not yet been fully elucidated, but it has been postulated that they are caused by impaired attentional and perceptual processes linked to degeneration in the cholinergic system [15–17]. A high Lewy body burden in extra-nigral cortical locations has been associated with both the development of hallucinations and dementia in pathological studies of Parkinson's disease [18–20]. The role of dopaminergic medication in precipitating hallucinations in PD is unclear. However, most cross-sectional and prospective longitudinal PD studies have failed to document dopaminergic medication dose as a determinant of hallucinations, so it may be that the dopaminergic system plays a role, but not in a direct causative way [16, 21].

Treatment

The primary form of hallucinations in PD needs to be distinguished from hallucinations as part of a delirium, and if hallucinations develop suddenly over hours or days in the setting of a neurodegenerative disorder, careful assessment for any physical cause of a delirium such as intercurrent infection, medication, electrolyte imbalance, hypoxemia, and alcohol and benzodiazepine withdrawal is warranted. Once these have been excluded, there are some low-cost pragmatic measures that can be adopted in a bid to alleviate the hallucinations. Improving lighting in the patient's direct environment and reducing visual triggers – if they exist – can be useful. Visual hallucinations are known to be more severe in dementing disease when visual acuity is poor [22]. Ophthalmological assessment may therefore sometimes be beneficial, to assess whether visual acuity can be improved with glasses or cataract surgery.

Pharmacological approaches to managing psychosis with hallucinations in Parkinson's disease can be challenging. A reduction of dopaminergic medication in some patients leads to an improvement in hallucinations, although reducing these medications may come at the cost of a deterioration in their motor disability. The currently available evidence supports the use of cholinesterase inhibitors such as rivastigmine in patients with PDD, as they can have a positive impact on hallucinations and help to stabilize cognition; however, additional research is needed to better establish their efficacy [23, 24]. The best evidence to date for treating hallucinations in PD is for clozapine, an atypical antipsychotic which has been shown to be efficacious at reducing hallucinations in PD in two randomized controlled trials [25, 26]. It has a favorable side effect profile in terms of having minimal impact on motor function but is generally not used by clinicians as a first-line treatment due to the need for relatively intense hematological monitoring to avoid the potentially serious complication of agranulocytosis. While quetiapine is frequently used to treat symptoms of PD psychosis in everyday practice, double-blind, placebo-controlled trials have demonstrated safety but not efficacy [27–29]. Recently, the selective serotonin 5-HT2A inverse agonist pimavanserin has shown promise for the treatment of hallucinations in PD in a phase III trial [30]. In future, a better understanding of the neuropathophysiology of hallucinations in PD should lead to improved therapeutic strategies for these patients.

References

1. Potter B. The tale of Jemima Puddle-Duck. London: Frederick Warne & Co.; 1908.
2. Postuma RB, Lang AE, Massicotte-Marquez J, Montplaisir J. Potential early markers of Parkinson disease in idiopathic REM sleep behavior disorder. Neurology. 2006;66:845–51.
3. McKeith IG, Galasko D, Kosaka K, Perry EK, Dickson DW, Hansen LA, Salmon DP, Lowe J, Mirra SS, Byrne EJ, Lennox G, Quinn NP, Edwardson JA, Ince PG, Bergeron C, Burns A, Miller BL, Lovestone S, Collerton D, Jansen EN, Ballard C, De Vos RA, Wilcock GK, Jelleinger KA, Perry RH. Consensus guidelines for the clinical and pathologic diagnosis of

dementia with Lewy bodies (DLB): report of the consortium on DLB international workshop. Neurology. 1996;47:1113–24.
4. Aarsland D, Litvan I, Salmon D, Galasko D, Wentzel-Larsen T, Larsen JP. Performance on the dementia rating scale in Parkinson's disease with dementia and dementia with Lewy bodies: comparison with progressive supranuclear palsy and Alzheimer's disease. J Neurol Neurosurg Psychiatry. 2003;74:1215–20.
5. Lippa CF, Duda JE, Grossman M, Hurtig HI, Aarsland D, Boeve BF, Brooks DJ, Dickson DW, Dubois B, Emre M, Fahn S, Farmer JM, Galasko D, Galvin JE, Goetz CG, Growdon JH, Gwinn-Hardy KA, Hardy J, Heutink P, Iwatsubo T, Kosaka K, Lee VM, Leverenz JB, Masliah E, McKeith IG, Nussbaum RL, Olanow CW, Ravina BM, Singleton AB, Tanner CM, Trojanowski JQ, Wszolek ZK, Group DPW. DLB and PDD boundary issues: diagnosis, treatment, molecular pathology, and biomarkers. Neurology. 2007;68:812–9.
6. Hely MA, Reid WG, Adena MA, Halliday GM, Morris JG. The Sydney multicenter study of Parkinson's disease: the inevitability of dementia at 20 years. Mov Disord. 2008;23:837–44.
7. Collerton D, Taylor JP. Advances in the treatment of visual hallucinations in neurodegenerative diseases. Futur Neurol. 2013;8:433–44.
8. Goetz CG, Fan W, Leurgans S, Bernard B, Stebbins GT. The malignant course of "benign hallucinations" in Parkinson disease. Arch Neurol. 2006;63:713–6.
9. Aarsland D, Larsen JP, Tandberg E, Laake K. Predictors of nursing home placement in Parkinson's disease: a population-based, prospective study. J Am Geriatr Soc. 2000;48:938–42.
10. Llebaria G, Pagonabarraga J, Martinez-Corral M, Garcia-Sanchez C, Pascual-Sedano B, Gironell A, Kulisevsky J. Neuropsychological correlates of mild to severe hallucinations in Parkinson's disease. Mov Disord. 2010;25:2785–91.
11. Barnes J, David AS. Visual hallucinations in Parkinson's disease: a review and phenomenological survey. J Neurol Neurosurg Psychiatry. 2001;70:727–33.
12. Zhu K, Van Hilten JJ, Putter H, Marinus J. Risk factors for hallucinations in Parkinson's disease: results from a large prospective cohort study. Mov Disord. 2013;28:755–62.
13. Comella CL, Tanner CM, Ristanovic RK. Polysomnographic sleep measures in Parkinson's disease patients with treatment-induced hallucinations. Ann Neurol. 1993;34:710–4.
14. Nomura T, Inoue Y, Mitani H, Kawahara R, Miyake M, Nakashima K. Visual hallucinations as REM sleep behavior disorders in patients with Parkinson's disease. Mov Disord. 2003;18:812–7.
15. Collerton D, Perry E, McKeith I. Why people see things that are not there: a novel perception and attention deficit model for recurrent complex visual hallucinations. Behav Brain Sci. 2005;28:737–57; discussion 757–94.
16. Fenelon G, Alves G. Epidemiology of psychosis in Parkinson's disease. J Neurol Sci. 2010;289:12.
17. Shine JM, Halliday GM, Naismith SL, Lewis SJ. Visual misperceptions and hallucinations in Parkinson's disease: dysfunction of attentional control networks? Mov Disord. 2011;26:2154–9.
18. Gallagher DA, Parkkinen L, O'Sullivan SS, Spratt A, Shah A, Davey CC, Bremner FD, Revesz T, Williams DR, Lees AJ, Schrag A. Testing an aetiological model of visual hallucinations in Parkinson's disease. Brain. 2011;134:3299–309.
19. Harding AJ, Broe GA, Halliday GM. Visual hallucinations in Lewy body disease relate to Lewy bodies in the temporal lobe. Brain. 2002;125:391–403.
20. Papapetropoulos S, McCorquodale DS, Gonzalez J, Jean-Gilles L, Mash DC. Cortical and amygdalar Lewy body burden in Parkinson's disease patients with visual hallucinations. Parkinsonism Relat Disord. 2006;12:253–6.
21. Merims D, Shabtai H, Korczyn AD, Peretz C, Weizman N, Giladi N. Antiparkinsonian medication is not a risk factor for the development of hallucinations in Parkinson's disease. J Transm. 2004;111:1447–53.

22. McShane R, Gedling K, Reading M, McDonald B, Esiri MM, Hope T. Prospective study of relations between cortical Lewy bodies, poor eyesight, and hallucinations in Alzheimer's disease. J Neurol Neurosurg Psychiatry. 1995;59:185–8.
23. Burn D, Emre M, McKeith I, De Deyn PP, Aarsland D, Hsu C, Lane R. Effects of rivastigmine in patients with and without visual hallucinations in dementia associated with Parkinson's disease. Mov Disord. 2006;21:1899–907.
24. Rolinski M, Fox C, Maidment I, McShane R. Cholinesterase inhibitors for dementia with Lewy bodies, Parkinson's disease dementia and cognitive impairment in Parkinson's disease. Cochrane Database Syst Rev. 2012;(3):CD006504.
25. Pollak P, Tison F, Rascol O, Destee A, Pere JJ, Senard JM, Durif F, Bourdeix I. Clozapine in drug induced psychosis in Parkinson's disease: a randomised, placebo controlled study with open follow up. J Neurol Neurosurg Psychiatry. 2004;75:689–95.
26. The Parkinson Study Group. Low-dose clozapine for the treatment of drug-induced psychosis in Parkinson's disease. N Engl J Med. 1999;340:757–63.
27. Rabey JM, Prokhorov T, Miniovitz A, Dobronevsky E, Klein C. Effect of quetiapine in psychotic Parkinson's disease patients: a double-blind labeled study of 3 months' duration. Mov Disord. 2007;22:313–8.
28. Shotbolt P, Samuel M, Fox C, David AS. A randomized controlled trial of quetiapine for psychosis in Parkinson's disease. Neuropsychiatr Dis Treat. 2009;5:327–32.
29. Kurlan R, Cummings J, Raman R, Thal L, Group, A. S. D. C. S. Quetiapine for agitation or psychosis in patients with dementia and parkinsonism. Neurology. 2007;68:1356–63.
30. Cummings J, Isaacson S, Mills R, Williams H, Chi-Burris K,Corbett A, Dhall R, Ballard C. Pimavanserin for patients with Parkinson's disease psychosis: a randomised, placebo-controlled phase 3 trial. Lancet. 2013. pii: S0140-6736(13)62106–6.

Chapter 10
Parkinsons and Parasomnias

Hugh Selsick

Mrs B is a 63-year-old married woman with a diagnosis of Parkinson's disease. Her symptoms started in her mid-50s and her symptoms gradually worsened over the subsequent years. However, she obtained satisfactory control of her daytime symptoms on gradually escalating doses of pramipexole which was divided into several smaller doses taken at intervals throughout the day. She was referred by her GP to the sleep disorders center for assessment of her "sleep disturbance."

She was initially seen in the sleep clinic with her husband. They gave very different accounts of what was troubling them. Mrs B complained of unrefreshing sleep and daytime sleepiness. Her Epworth Sleepiness Score (ESS) was 14/24. The ESS is a questionnaire that asks the patient about the likelihood of falling asleep in eight different scenarios, and an ESS greater than 11 is indicative of excessive daytime sleepiness. Mrs B attributed her sleepiness to the side effects of her medication. On a typical night, she would go to bed at 10:00 p.m. and would be asleep within minutes. Subjectively, she would sleep through to 7:30 a.m. when her husband would wake her to give her the first dose of medication. She would be almost completely unable to move on waking due to the Parkinson's symptoms and would go back to sleep for a further 2 h while the medication took effect. She would then have a number of brief naps during the day. These were all unplanned as she would fall asleep watching TV, in the car, etc.

Her husband presented a very different history. He complained that Mrs B was having extended episodes of crying during the night. These episodes typically started at around 1:00 a.m. and could last anything from a few minutes to several hours. She was generally unresponsive during these episodes and was not consolable. During the episodes, her eyes were closed and the crying was not associated with any body movements. This picture was confirmed by a video of one of the

H. Selsick, MBBCh, BSC (Hon)
University College London Hospitals, Insomnia Clinic, Royal London Hospital for Integrated Medicine, London, UK
e-mail: hugh.selsick@uclh.nhs.uk

J. Priller, H. Rickards (eds.), *Neuropsychiatry Case Studies*,
DOI 10.1007/978-3-319-42190-2_10

episodes that Mr B recorded on his mobile phone. Mrs B had no recollection of these episodes and did not report having particularly distressing dreams. The episodes had started about 3 years before and had been getting progressively worse. Mr B initially thought she might be experiencing pain as, at the time the episodes started, Mrs B was experiencing severe sciatica. However, Mrs B had injections for the sciatica which effectively controlled the pain, but the episodes continued. Mr B therefore surmised that she was responding to distressing dreams; Mrs B agreed with this though she could not recall what the dreams were. The episodes never happened during daytime naps, though this was attributed to the fact that the naps were rarely longer than a few minutes.

Mr B had taken to sleeping in a different room on most nights as the crying was disrupting his sleep and impacting on his work.

Background History

Mrs B had a relatively unremarkable history prior to the onset of the Parkinson's disease. She had been happily married to Mr B since her early 20s and had two sons by normal vaginal delivery. She had no history of psychological trauma and no history of head injury. She had chronic lower back pain due to degeneration of the facet joints in her lumbar spine. She had been on antidepressants on and off since receiving the diagnosis of Parkinson's disease and at the time of presentation had been on Sertraline 100 mg for 2 years. She had an adverse reaction to opiate analgesics. Her medication regime was:

07:30 – Pramipexole 1050 mcg + Sertraline 100 mg
11:00 – Pramipexole 350 mcg
15:00 – Pramipexole 350 mcg
19:00 – Pramipexole 350 mcg

Examination

The initial examination was done in the late morning once the medication had taken effect. She did not have any resting tremor and had no discernible rigidity. Her walking and speech were largely unaffected. The only noticeable daytime sign of the Parkinson's disease was a mask-like facies. Her reflexes were normal and the rest of her physical examination was unremarkable.

On mental state examination, she was alert and well oriented to time and place. Her mood was good with an appropriate and reactive affect. Thoughts were normal in form and content. Cognition was not formally assessed as this was being monitored by her neurology team, and there was no indication of any cognitive deficit.

Differential Diagnosis

The first disorder that sprung to mind was a rapid eye movement (REM) sleep behavior disorder or RBD. During REM sleep, there is complete atonia of all skeletal muscles with the exception of muscles in the middle ear, orbit of the eye, and the diaphragm. This atonia prevents motor signals generated during dreaming from reaching the muscles and therefore prevents dream enactment during REM. RBD is the loss of this normal atonia, and it leads to a range of behaviors during REM sleep. These include crying, shouting, running movements, punching, and throwing oneself out of bed. It is extremely common in Parkinson's disease; indeed it is often the first sign and may precede the onset of daytime motor symptoms by many years.

However, it is unusual for RBD to last for most of the night as occurred with Mrs B. It is more likely to occur in discrete episodes concentrated in the second half of the night when the majority of REM sleep occurs. Episodes that occur in the first half of the night are more likely to emerge from slow-wave sleep (SWS) which is the deepest stage of sleep. SWS parasomnias include sleepwalking, night terrors, and confusional arousals. It is also not uncommon for there to be a combination of SWS and REM parasomnias, and so it was thought that this may be the case with Mrs B.

The other potential diagnosis was an unusual form of epilepsy. Nocturnal epilepsy is usually characterized by stereotypical movements rather than crying but unlike parasomnias can present with multiple episodes throughout the night as was the case with Mrs B.

Initial Investigations

Mrs B was admitted for an overnight polysomnogram with extended montage. This investigation includes an electroencephalogram (EEG) and an electrooculogram (EOG) to detect and stage sleep and look for epileptic phenomena, chin and anterior tibialis electromyogram to monitor muscle tone and detect subtle limb movements, an ECG, oximetry, and a video camera. Recording started in the mid afternoon and continued overnight.

Mrs B had a number of brief naps during the afternoon and evening, none lasting more than a few minutes, and in all cases she experienced only stage 1 and stage 2 (light) sleep. No unusual behaviors were noted. No epileptic phenomena were detected during wakefulness or sleep.

Lights out was at 11:00 p.m. and Mrs B fell asleep within 2 min. She had severe periodic limb movements of sleep which were detected on the tibialis EMG but were obvious enough to be picked up on the video as well. However, these did not lead to many arousals. At around 1:00 a.m., Mrs B started crying and whimpering. On examination of the EEG, she was awake during this episode. After 25 min, she fell asleep again. An hour later, she had a more prolonged period of crying, and, once again, the EEG showed she was awake. Her eyes were closed on both occasions, and there were no associated limb movements. No REM sleep was recorded (possibly due to the REM suppressing effects of the Sertraline), and therefore it was impossible to determine if there was any RBD.

Her respiration was entirely normal during the night, and no epileptiform activity was detected.

Progress

The results of the study were discussed with Mrs B at her next clinic appointment. It was explained to her that the crying episodes occurred when she was awake. To our surprise, she immediately agreed with the results. She explained that since we had started investigating the episodes, she had become more aware of them. She said she would awaken during the night, usually due to the need to pass water, to find that her Parkinson's medication had worn off. She was completely immobilized by the Parkinson's and was therefore unable to move or talk. She would start crying and whimpering, partly due to her distress and partly to try to alert her husband. She would then drift in and out of sleep for the rest of the night, experiencing the immobilization and consequent distress on each awakening. Eventually, she would be so fatigued that she would fall into a deep sleep an hour or two before her husband gave her the medication.

We therefore wrote to her neurologists to ask them to consider either increasing her pramipexole or increasing the gap between daytime doses so she could take her last dose right before bedtime. They agreed to both strategies and changed her medication regime to:

07:30 – Pramipexole 1,050 mcg + Sertraline 100 mg
12:00 – Pramipexole 350 mcg
18:00 – Pramipexole 350 mcg
22:00 – Pramipexole 700 mcg

At the next appointment, Mrs B reported a significant improvement in her symptoms. She was still waking twice a night but was able to move with relative ease. She would then go to the bathroom and return to sleep quickly. The crying episodes had abated completely and her daytime sleepiness had resolved. Her Epworth Sleepiness Score was 6/24. Mr B was also very pleased with her progress, and, as she was no longer disrupting his sleep, they had started sleeping in the same bed again.

Further Investigation

Mrs B had been booked for a repeat PSG in the hope of getting an episode of REM sleep in order to determine whether there was any RBD. However, once the medication had been changed, there were no residual behaviors that might lead to a clinical suspicion of RBD, and so the PSG was canceled.

Diagnosis

Mrs B was experiencing severe muscle rigidity due to the effects of her medication wearing off. This was disrupting her sleep and causing significant daytime fatigue. She was initially unaware of the nocturnal awakenings, probably due to the severe fatigue and the repeated cycling between wakefulness and sleep.

What Did I Learn from This Case?

The most important lesson I learned from Mrs B is that not everything that occurs during the sleep period is a sleep disorder. We spend approximately a third of our lives sleeping, and therefore it should not be surprising that many conditions will occur during the sleep period. Furthermore, a patient's self-reported state of wakefulness or sleep may not always be accurate. It is common for patients to believe they are awake when they are in fact asleep. This is known as paradoxical insomnia or sleep state misperception. However, it is also possible to have the opposite effect where the patient feels they are asleep when they are in fact awake. This is more likely to occur when the patient is drowsy or is repeatedly cycling between wakefulness and sleep as often occurs in obstructive sleep apnea. Head banging, rocking, and eating, for example, can all occur during sleep but have also been described in awake patients though these patients have no memory of the events and therefore presume they occurred during sleep. These cases demonstrate the importance of the PSG in diagnosing and managing sleep disorders.

The other issue raised by this case is a more general one. Our sleep period is not only a time when we experience a very different physiological and mental state, but it is also the longest period during the day when we do not eat, drink, or take medication. When medication is given more than once a day, it is often timed to be evenly distributed across the waking hours rather than across the whole 24 h. Thus, a three times daily medication is usually given at breakfast, lunch, and dinner. There is then a gap of up to 12 h before the next morning dose is taken. This is clearly done as a matter of convenience, and in many cases it is not problematic. However, as this case shows, there are circumstances when the nighttime medication gap can lead to significant difficulties. Thus, it is important when prescribing to be aware of the potential for symptoms to emerge when drug levels are low.

Chapter 11
The Possible Talents of Tourette Syndrome

Andrea E. Cavanna

Y.B. and O.B. are two brothers who were referred to the specialist Tourette syndrome clinic at the age of 9 and 18, respectively. Beyond apparent similarities, their clinical presentations revealed intriguing and challenging differences, which illustrate the intrinsic variety of the "compulsivity-impulsivity" spectrum characterizing the behavioral side of Tourette syndrome.

Clinical Presentations

Y.B.'s tics first appeared when he was 5 years old. His motor tics included mouth opening, shirt pulling, trouser pulling, neck extension, stamping, eye blinking, eye rolling, and other postural tics (standing up in particular positions). Phonic tics were in the form of sounds at different pitches, and there was a history of echolalia. A particularly troublesome tic at the time of assessment was spitting, especially on toilet seats and sleeves: since Y.B. had to wipe his mouth after this tic, this occasionally caused abrasions around his oral region. His mother noticed that the mouth opening tic could also occur at night, but this had reduced since commencing antidopaminergic medication. The tics were characteristically preceded by premonitory urges and tended to follow a

A.E. Cavanna, MD, PhD
Department of Neuropsychiatry, The Barberry National Centre for Mental Health, Birmingham, UK
e-mail: andrea.cavanna@bsmhft.nhs.uk

J. Priller, H. Rickards (eds.), *Neuropsychiatry Case Studies*,
DOI 10.1007/978-3-319-42190-2_11

waxing and waning course over time. He scored 78 % on the Tourette syndrome diagnostic confidence index and 43 % on the Yale Global Tic Severity Scale, indicating moderate tic severity. Y.B.'s mother described him as very active and fidgety since early childhood; moreover, she recalled behaviors where he would sometimes line things up at home in a particular order and arrange and clear up toys with particular emphasis on symmetry ("evening-up" behaviors). Overall, his obsessive-compulsive behaviors (OCBs) were of mild severity, despite a clear-cut anxiety-driven tendency to compulsive repetitions. Y.B. was also described as overly self-critical when doing practical work. School reports were highly positive both academically and with regard to his behavior. He was described as very sociable and talented.

During his consultation, both Y.B. and his mother reported excessive sedation as a possible side effect of his anti-tic medication. By changing his antidopaminergic medication (the atypical aripiprazole in place of the neuroleptic haloperidol), his sedation improved, and his creativity found full expression, as shown in his original poetry production (Fig. 11.1).

THE MAD GUY POEM

Once upon a time
A guy spent a dime
He went to a shop
With a humongous hop
He saw a army man
With a hand made fan
He bought a water gun
And had so much fun

He jumped
And bumped
His head
on a Bed
Hanging from the ceiling
he had a bad feeling
He froze in mid air
And saw an awesome fair
He jumped out of the air
Like a bundle of hair

He rushed
With no trust
And bump
he had a big lump
It was card board
He pulled a cord
Went to court and
And thought
Am I dead
"No" im in bed

THE END

aged 9
23/05/2011

Fig. 11.1 Talented creativity in the context of Tourette syndrome: poetry sample from Y.B., aged 9

Family history was unremarkable for tic symptoms, apart from his older brother. His paternal grandfather was reported to have obsessive-compulsive symptoms.

When O.B. was referred to the specialist Tourette syndrome clinic, he already had an 11-year history of tics. His first tic at the age of 7 was mouth opening. He subsequently developed multiple motor tics affecting his whole body. These included raising eyebrows, eye blinking, eye winking, rolling the eyes up, looking sideways, movements of the lips, swallowing, smiling, teeth grinding, teeth gnashing, spitting, smelling, licking things, blowing, head nodding, head turning, neck stretching, shoulder shrugging, arms flexing and extending, finger drumming, leg flexing and extending, kicking, toe movements, whole-body movements, adjusting clothes, looking in mirrors, stamping, hopping, squatting, turning, bending, hitting, pinching, touching, and tapping body parts. His vocal tics included grunting, throat clearing, snorting, whooping, sniffing, humming, squeaking, hissing, growling, gasping, clicking, yelping, noisy breathing, whistling, and coughing. In addition to simple tics, O.B. presented with complex motor and vocal tics, including echolalia, echopraxia, palilalia, palipraxia, coprolalia, and copropraxia. His tics had characteristic premonitory urges, and he was able to voluntarily suppress them at the expense of a subsequent rebound in tic severity. He scored 100 % on the Tourette syndrome diagnostic confidence index and 65 % on the Yale Global Tic Severity Scale, indicating marked tic severity. Like his younger brother, he presented with a repertoire of OCBs, which were severe enough to cause significant distress and functional impairment, leading to a concomitant diagnosis of obsessive-compulsive disorder (OCD). Specifically, he reported experiencing obsessional thoughts and performing counting rituals; however, it was clear that in his case, the comorbid OCD tended to result in more impulsive actions, such as bilateral kicking, which was associated with arithmomania (obsessional counting). This repetitive movement was most apparent when walking and caused marked shoe damage, particularly at the shoe tip. Notably, it was not present when sitting or lying. The frequency and severity of this repetitive movement resulted in a considerable extent of shoe deterioration and associated hip and toe pain (Fig. 11.2).

The impulsive-compulsive nature of this repetitive movement was further suggested by its refractoriness to conventional antidopaminergic treatment and partial response to serotonergic medication [1]. In social settings, O.B. found himself at risk of performing actions that were poorly conceived, prematurely expressed, unduly risky, or inappropriate to the situation and that could potentially result in undesirable outcomes. O.B. was able to overcome the difficulties related to his severe symptoms and developed self-confidence and motivation to successfully engage in both social and work activities.

Discussion

Tourette syndrome is a clinical diagnosis based on the chronic presence of multiple motor tics and at least one vocal or phonic tic since childhood. Further investigations, including liver function tests, serum copper, and ceruloplasmin to exclude

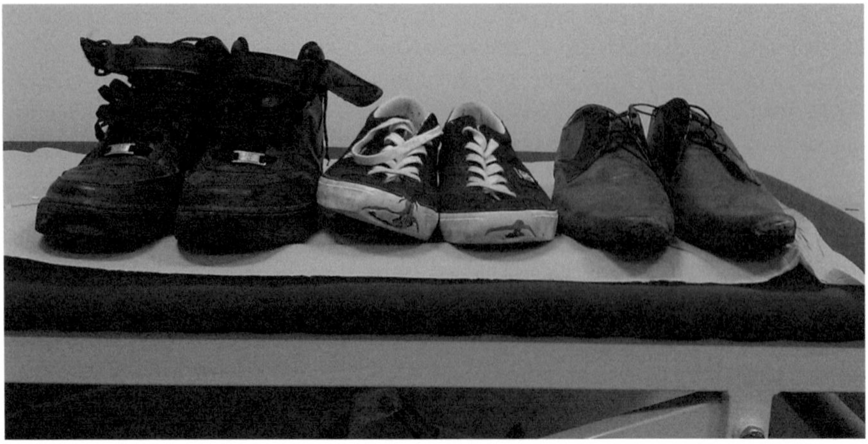

Fig. 11.2 Repetitive kicking resulting in bilateral shoe deterioration in O.B., aged 19

Wilson disease, blood film for neuroacanthocytosis, neuroimaging for suspected stroke or other brain lesions, and neurophysiology for suspected epilepsy (e.g., myoclonic epilepsy or absences resembling staring tics), are warranted in case of atypical presentations. These can include unusual types of tics, such as isolated dystonic tics, or unusual clinical histories, such as acute onset of tics and/or late onset in adulthood. The clinical presentations of the two brothers were characteristic and did not require further investigations. What can be more challenging is the assessment of the behavioral symptoms associated with Tourette syndrome. It is now well recognized that about 90 % of patients with Tourette syndrome present with at least one comorbid condition, both in specialist centers and in the community. The most common comorbidities are OCD, attention-deficit hyperactivity disorder (ADHD), affective disorders, and impulse control disorders [2]. These psychiatric comorbidities are often more important than tics themselves in affecting health-related quality of life for patients with Tourette syndrome [3].

What Did I Learn from These Cases?

I learned two main lessons from looking after these brothers. I learned that the clinical phenotype of Tourette syndrome can present with subtle yet important differences even within first-degree relatives, resulting in different presentations and requiring different management approaches. Interestingly, although both brothers presented with behavioral symptoms in association with tics, their behavioral repertoires sit at the opposite ends of the "compulsivity-impulsivity" spectrum [4]. The tics which characterize Tourette syndrome can be accompanied by repetitive behaviors that are performed according to certain rules or in a stereotypical fashion (as in Y.B.'s case) or a predisposition toward rapid, unplanned reactions to internal or external stimuli without regard to their potentially harmful consequences (as in O.B.'s case). I also learned that Tourette syndrome can be inspirational in several ways. Firstly, if appropriately channeled, the so-called blind force of the subcortex characterizing Tourette syndrome can result in talent and creativity, which should possibly be spared when using pharmacotherapy to treat tics [5]. Secondly, the remarkable achievements of persons with tics – despite their often severe symptoms – should never stop being a source of inspiration for anyone who has the privilege to get to know them.

References

1. Mitchell JW, Cavanna AE. Bilateral shoe deterioration as a result of complex motor tics in Tourette syndrome. J Neuropsychiatry Clin Neurosci. 2014;26(2):E22–3.
2. Cavanna AE, Rickards HE. The psychopathological spectrum of Gilles de la Tourette syndrome. Neurosci Biobehav Rev. 2013;37:1008–15.
3. Eddy CM, Cavanna AE, Gulisano M, Calì P, Robertson MM, Rizzo R. The effects of comorbid obsessive-compulsive disorders and attention-deficit hyperactivity disorder on quality of life in Tourette syndrome. J Neuropsychiatry Clin Neurosci. 2012;24:458–62.
4. Wright A, Rickards H, Cavanna AE. Impulse control disorders in Gilles de la Tourette syndrome. J Neuropsychiatry Clin Neurosci. 2012;24:16–27.
5. Sacks O. Tourette's syndrome and creativity. BMJ. 1992;305:1515–6.

Chapter 12
On the Nature of Separation Challenges and Attachment Solutions in Severe, Refractory Gilles de la Tourette Syndrome (GTS): Deep Brain Stimulation (DBS) Has Been Helpful, But What About Rikki and Luci and Now Riley?

James F. Leckman

Steve is a 58-year-old male with a lifelong history of severe GTS, which has resulted in permanent injury to his cervical spine and spinal cord secondary to chronic and forceful head-snapping tics. His injuries have left him nearly paralyzed on his left side. Both his grip and arm strength are markedly diminished in his (dominant) left hand. In the past, the weakness in his left ankle has necessitated the use of an ankle brace.

Background History

Steve has had a lifelong course of GTS beginning at the age of 3 years. He has facial, head and neck, and vocal tics. His head-snapping tics are particularly forceful and severe. His vocal tics have included grunting, loud noises, and cursing at times. He was diagnosed with GTS at the age of 13 years by Arthur Shapiro. Dr. Shapiro was one of the very first clinical investigators to devote a substantial portion of his career to the clinical care of individuals with GTS while simultaneously collecting systematic data from a large cohort (>500) of individuals with GTS in the hope that his data would "… help to mitigate the potentially horrendous consequences of their illness by correcting some of the myths and fallacies that have haunted patients for centuries" [1, 2]. Dr. Shapiro started Steve on haloperidol at an average daily dose of 6–10 mg. In 1976, he participated in trials of a number of other medications including a formal clozapine trial at the Clinical Center at the National Institutes of Health in Bethesda, Maryland, in an attempt to control his tics.

J.F. Leckman, MD, PhD
Yale School of Medicine, Child Study Center, New Haven, CT, USA
e-mail: james.leckman@yale.edu

J. Priller, H. Rickards (eds.), *Neuropsychiatry Case Studies*,
DOI 10.1007/978-3-319-42190-2_12

Steve has been followed at the Yale Child Study Center at Yale University since 1996. At the time I first met Steve, he was working full-time as an emergency medical technician. He was married, but over time, his relationship with his wife became more and more problematic that was due in part to his tic symptoms and the fact that they both had very demanding and not well-aligned work schedules. Eventually, his marriage ended, and he became increasingly reliant on his younger brother. Although Steve has excellent social skills with many friends and colleagues, he was lonely and became progressively depressed.

During the ensuing years, I initiated a number of additional medication trials in an effort to control his tics (haloperidol, pimozide, risperidone, clonidine, pergolide, and clonazepam) and to treat his obsessive-compulsive disorder (OCD) and depression (fluoxetine). When Steve was not working or on call, he reported that smoking marijuana helped him to relax and that he had fewer tics during and after smoking a joint.

Despite the marijuana and high doses of anti-tic medications, his self-injurious tics continued to worsen his cervical myelopathy involving primarily the left upper and left lower extremities to a point that he was no longer able to use his previously dominant left arm. Steve was referred for a multilevel laminectomy for cervical cord decompression. However, because of fear that Steve's persistent tics would further exacerbate his cervical injury, if a fixation was performed, only a decompression procedure was performed.

In 2004, after watching a television program that presented a GTS patient being "cured" by deep brain stimulation (DBS), Steve contacted me and expressed a strong interest in having the surgery. At that time, his tics were occurring in all settings and comprised frequent, forceful, violent head jerking, slamming his forearms against his forehead, throwing his elbows against his ribs, abdominal tensing, and leg tics. His most worrisome tic involved a severe head "snapping" in which he would thrust his head down flexing his cervical spine and then violently "snap" his head back over his shoulder in an extreme and painful extension of his cervical spine. His vocal tics included grunting, screeching, a goose-like noise, and occasional swearing. He also described the need to repeat activities, line things up, touch corners, and the urge to touch hot objects.

Examination

Examination revealed neck painful to touch and marked spasm of the paraspinal muscles on palpation. Range of motion of his neck was normal with regard to flexion and extension; however, there was difficulty with lateral rotation and flexion particularly on the left side. Tone was decreased in upper extremities and increased in lower extremities. Deep tendon reflexes were brisk bilaterally on upper extremities and 3+ bilaterally in lower extremities. He had unsustained clonus on both sides and a positive Babinski bilaterally. There was reduced pinprick sensation at C5 and C6 on left. At that time, on mental status examination, Steve was depressed and obtunded from the high doses of neuroleptics, pain medications, and marijuana. He was confined to a wheelchair due to left-sided weakness and in a state of near-total mental and physical disability.

Initial Investigations

MRI of his cervical spine revealed congenital spinal stenosis with superimposed severe stenosis from C3 to C7, myelomalacia, and atrophy.

Initial DBS Surgery

Because of Steve's refractory tics and progressive neurological injury, he underwent his first DBS electrode placement in July 2004. At this time, two Medtronic quadripolar deep brain stimulating electrodes were placed in the medial part of the thalamus. His tics were markedly improved (virtually no motor tics reported by the patient and his family) for 2 weeks immediately following the surgery. During this time, his stimulator remained off. Approximately 6 weeks following the surgery, his tics returned in forceful bouts. Adjustments were frequently made to his neural stimulator, and nearly 20 programming sessions were conducted over a 2-year period. The frequency of the stimulation was stable at 130 Hz, and the pulse width varied between 60 and 120 μs. The final settings for the stimulation amplitude (volts) were 2.0 (left), 2.0 (right), bilateral stimulation frequency of 130 Hz, and bilateral pulse width of 90 μs with the electrode settings at 1−, 3+ on the left and 5−, 7+ on the right. When the voltage was increased too much, Steve consistently reported an unpleasant "woozy" feeling but denied any other side effects.

Over the next several years, Steve spoke with me nearly every morning to provide brief updates. We kept a running log of the number of tics he had each day. During these conversations, in addition to providing his "tic count," Steve almost invariably spoke about his support staff and about his dogs Luci and Rikki. Slowly I began to realize how close his emotional ties were to Luci and Rikki.

Over time he was gradually able to tolerate the voltage increases. Two years after the surgery, he estimated a 95 % improvement in the frequency of his tics. Although the number and frequency of his tics markedly diminished, there was only a mild decrease in the forcefulness of his tics. His severe head-snapping tic, although less frequent, had not improved in forcefulness. His dosage of haloperidol was reduced from 6 mg per day to 1 mg per day. His obsessive-compulsive symptoms were also improved. Despite the improvements in his tics, OC symptoms, and mood, his neurological status continued to worsen, albeit more slowly than before the surgery. Due to his continued tics and persistent pain, he received botulinum toxin injections into the splenius capitis and trapezius muscles at 13, 16, and 20 months postsurgery. There was only minimal reported benefit (some decreased pain and stiffness in his right shoulder). His neck pain and headaches, however, remained unchanged, and the botulinum toxin injections were discontinued in March 2006.

Despite the marked reduction in the frequency of his tics, the forcefulness of his tics remained high, and he continued to experience neurological damage to his spine because of head snapping. For these reasons, 4 years after the first operation, a second set of DBS electrodes was placed in the sensorimotor portion of the internal segment of the globus pallidus pars interna (GPi) in 2009. The programming of these electrodes began approximately 1 month after the surgery, using a set of parameters similar to those used in the treatment of dystonia. With the continued programming of both sets of the electrodes, both the frequency and forcefulness of his tics decreased, and his daily tic count was in the range of 0–100 (average 50). Indeed, on December 20, 2009, Steve experienced his first "tic-free" day in his living memory. It was a time to celebrate with Luci, Rikki, and me. At that time, his GPi leads were turned off. Bilaterally, his thalamic settings were a frequency of 130 Hz, a pulse width of 90 s, and an amplitude of 2.0 V. The contact points were left (1−, 3) and right (5−, 7). More recently, we again turned his GPi leads on, but then he experienced a failure of his GPi leads due in part to his severe head-snapping tic that caused a malfunction of the wires connecting the electrodes to the stimulator. In addition, his thalamic electrodes have been turned off for more than a year without any marked change in the frequency or forcefulness of his tics. Most recently, Steve has requested that he had the stimulator replaced for his thalamic electrodes.

Most Recent Examination

Due to Steve's disability, he has made relatively few trips to New Haven in the past few years. On two occasions, however, clinicians and research assistants have traveled to his home. The photograph (Fig. 12.1) is from their first visit. Rikki and Luci are on the couch next to Steve.

During my most recent trip to visit Steve, I had the opportunity to meet Riley. During that conversation and in preparation for drafting this case report, Steve expressed again in an emotionally compelling way, how when he lies in bed with Riley next to him; he has "no tics." He is able to "relax" completely and even his neck pain "goes away." As with Luci and Rikki in the past, Riley is now Steve's constant companion.

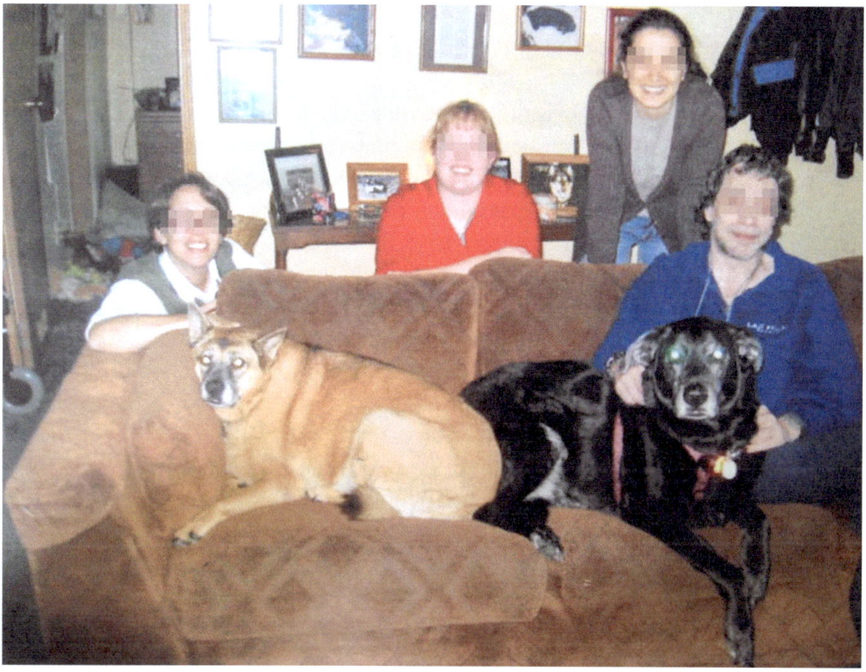

Fig. 12.1 Steve; Luci; Rikki; Angelica Landeros-Weisenberger, MD; Megan Smith, MD; and Maria Motlagh, MD (Note: Edited portions of the text first appeared in: Bajwa et al. [6] and Motlagh et al. [4])

What Did I Learn from This Case?

The healing presence and close emotional attachment of Steve to his dogs and their reciprocal attachment to him are among the most effective interventions for tics that Steve has at this point in his life. Steve's frequent telephone calls and brief conversations with me, in my opinion, are also manifestations of his attachment solution to the separation challenges posed by GTS. Gregory Fricchione's compassionate and scholarly review of the likely evolutionary origins and complex neurobiology of human attachment is compelling and should be a "must read" for individuals considering a career in the field of medicine. Fricchione encourages us as clinicians to provide compassionate humanistic and longitudinal care as it is the foundation for the physical, emotional, and spiritual healing of our patients.

Steve is not alone. Many individuals with GTS struggle to make lasting interpersonal attachments, and many echo Steve's genuine solace when being with "his girls." I can think of several other "friends" and patients with severe lifelong GTS who struggle with the social ostracism and at times social phobia that GTS can bring in its wake. Other patients and their families often have attachment solutions with romantic partners, but their long-term attachment to their clinicians is also critically important for their well-being, even if a "cure" is not at hand. "Abe" and his relationship with Donald J. Cohen comes to mind [3]. I first met Abe when he was tied to bed on a pediatric ward because of severe hitting tics that eventually led to the destruction of Abe's nasal cartilage so that his nose was just a flap of skin on his face. Despite Abe's severe, lifelong self-injurious tics, Donald Cohen through his close interpersonal and compassionate care kept Abe's development on track and fostered Abe's sense that through "drive, desire, and willpower," he could overcome his tics. The outcome is that Abe is socially adept and able to maintain part-time employment despite his disabling tics and, perhaps most important, Abe has been able to maintain a close romantic relationship with "Karen," his partner for more than 15 years. Abe exemplifies what it means to "accept" his GTS (watch http://tsa-usa.org/ZHBO/VideoPlayer.html).

The DBS surgery was lifesaving for Steve. I only wish DBS was as beneficial for all the individuals with GTS. Ideally, we would know precisely where the most efficacious anatomical target was located and what the optimum stimulator settings would be [4]. Sadly, some of our patients have had no benefit whatsoever even after repeated surgeries. Others have had serious infections either postoperatively or as a result of hitting the incision sites or causing inflammation along the track of the wires running between the stimulator implanted in their chest and the sites in the skull where the electrodes have been placed.

I also wish we had ideal anti-tic medications, but we do not. It may be that compounds such as fatty acid amide hydrolase (FAAH) inhibitors will prove to be beneficial as FAAH inhibitors enhance the endogenous cannabinoids without causing a "high." There are several lines of evidence that cannabinoids may be effective in the treatment of tic disorders [5], and many of the severe GTS cases that I follow rely on smoking marijuana and cannabinoid derivatives. Indeed, several families have relocated to ensure access to medical marijuana.

Finally, although GTS is both phenomenologically and etiologically heterogenous, I am convinced that neuroimmunological interventions may in the future hold real promise for therapeutic benefit. Based on the whole transcriptome analyses of the caudate nuclei and putamen of nine individuals with GTS vs. nine matched "controls" that was recently completed in Flora Vaccarino's laboratory at Yale, it is clear that what we call "the immune system" may well be an important contributor to normal brain development and function as well as to the pathobiology of this enigmatic condition. I am hopeful that as we gain a greater understanding of the immune system, novel compounds will emerge that will provide a therapeutic benefit for GTS as well as a broad range of other neuropsychiatric and neurodegenerative disorders. My favorite cells, at present, are the microglia traditionally seen as the resident macrophages of the brain; it is now clear that they play a crucial role in brain development and circuit formation.

Finally, I should mention that over time as new knowledge has emerged, I have come to appreciate the sheer and utter complexity of brain function. Indeed, I often now find myself saying, the more I learn, the less I truly understand about how our brains develop and function moment-to-moment. It is also clear how important our interactions and relationships are with others (pets included) in this ever-changing world. I am also convinced that our relationships can have a direct impact on our well-being as well as our physical and neuropsychiatric health. This is a lesson I have learned, in part from Steve, Luci, Rikki, and Riley. Thanks as well to my many colleagues who have played important roles in my care for Steve including Donald J. Cohen, Maria G. Motlagh, Angeli Landeros-Weisenberger, Megan E. Smith, Robert A. King, Joan Miravite (DBS programmer par excellence), and Alain C. J. de Lotbinière (a gifted neurosurgeon).

References

1. Shapiro AK, Shapiro ES, Bruun RD, Sweet RD. Gilles de la Tourette syndrome. New York: Raven press; 1978.
2. Shapiro AK, Shapiro ES, Young JG, Feinberg TE. Gilles de la Tourette syndrome. 2nd ed. New York: Raven press; 1988, 584 pp.
3. Cohen DJ, Leckman JF. Introduction: the self under siege. In: Leckman JF, Cohen DJ, editors. Tourette's syndrome: tics, obsessions, compulsions – developmental psychopathology and clinical care. New York: Wiley; 1998. p. 11–4.
4. Motlagh MG, Smith ME, Landeros-Weisenberger A, Kobets AJ, King RA, Miravite J, de Lotbinière, ACJ, Alterman RL, Mogilner AY, Pourfar, MH, Okun, MS, Leckman JF. Lessons learned from open label deep brain stimulation for Tourette syndrome: 8 cases over 7 years. Tremor Other Hyperkinetic Mov. 2013;3. pii: tre-03-170-4428-1.
5. Müller-Vahl KR. Treatment of Tourette syndrome with cannabinoids. Behav Neurol. 2013;27(1):119–24.

Bibliography

Bajwa RJ, de Lotbinière AJ, King RA, Jabbari B, Kunze K, Quatrano S, Scahill L, Leckman JF. Brief report: deep brain stimulation in Tourette's syndrome. Mov Disord. 2007;22(9):1346–50.

Fricchione GL. Compassion and healing in medicine and society: on the nature and use of attachment solutions to separation challenges. Baltimore: Johns Hopkins University Press; 2011.

Leckman JF. What does immunology have to do with brain development and psychopathology? J Child Psychol Psychiatry. 2014;55(6):632–4.

Lennington JB, Coppola G, Kataoka-Sasaki Y, Fernandez T, Palejev D, Li Y, Huttner A, Pletikos M, Šestan N, Leckman JF, Vaccarino FM. Transcriptome analysis of the human striatum in Tourette syndrome. Biol Psychiatry. 2014;79(5):372–82.

Martino D. Immunity and stress response in Tourette syndrome. In: Martino D, Leckman JF, editors. Tourette syndrome. New York: Oxford University Press; 2013. p. 301–28.

Chapter 13
Paroxysmal Disorders in Autism: Problems with Diagnosis and Management

Kanu Achinivu

Paroxysmal events are common in the autistic population and come in a variety of forms including seizures, repetitive behaviors, aggressive behaviors, sensory perception problems, hyperactive behaviors, inattention, and impulsivity. Diagnosis can be challenging, especially in the learning disabled population. A typical challenging case is presented.

DM is a 24-year-old man who has a diagnosis of autism and severe learning disability as well as bipolar disorder and was referred for assessment due to behavioral problems; he was demonstrating at his residential placement where he had moved into the previous 6 months from the family home. Concerns were raised as he was showing "increase in behavioral difficulty" with a request to rule out a tic disorder. Behavioral problems included possible "seizures"; unpredictable aggressive behavior; restless agitation; mood swings; short attention span; sleep disturbance; complex behaviors comprising of whole body movements such as turning and twirling at a particular spot; complex shoulder movements; vocalizations such as repeated throat clearing, echolalia, and coprolalia; and fascination with water.

He was on a variety of prescribed medications including sodium valproate at a dose of 2.4 g a day, carbamazepine at a dose of 1 g a day, risperidone at a dose of 4 mg daily, aripiprazole at a dose of 20 mg daily, and quetiapine XR at a dose of 100 mg a day and a variety of gastrointestinal medications.

K. Achinivu, MBBS, MSc, MRCPsych
Department of Neuropsychiatry, National Centre for Mental Health, The Barberry, Birmingham, UK
e-mail: kanu.achinivu@bsmhft.nhs.uk

J. Priller, H. Rickards (eds.), *Neuropsychiatry Case Studies*,
DOI 10.1007/978-3-319-42190-2_13

Background History

DM is the eldest of two boys; the other also has a diagnosis of autism. There is also a history of epilepsy in a cousin and bipolar disorder in an aunt.

He was born following an apparent normal pregnancy and delivery and seemed to be developing normally until the age of 18 months when his parents became concerned about the lack of appropriate speech development. He was initially seen by a speech therapist who recommended a referral to specialist services. Following assessment, local child psychiatry services made a diagnosis of autism at the age of 3. This diagnosis enabled him to access specialist interventions including play therapy, speech and language therapy, and psychology and psychiatry input.

Behavioral problems existed from an early age though were always manageable. These included inattention, intermittently disturbed sleep suggestive of a delayed sleep phase syndrome, hyperactivity, impulsivity, and simple motor tics. Later on, complex motor tics and vocal tics became apparent. This led to the introduction of antipsychotic medication. Around the age of 9, "challenging" behaviors developed with head banging, "broodiness," increased arousal and agitation, anxiety, emotional instability, hyperactivity, restlessness, unpredictable aggression, and self-injury. There was no history of a sustained mood state suggestive of a primary mood disorder. A diagnosis of bipolar disorder was made a year later, and DM was commenced on sodium valproate and risperidone for mood regulation and anti-aggression effect. This had minimal effect on DM's behavior.

On attaining adulthood, further changes to medication were made with the introduction of carbamazepine and reduction of risperidone with no significant benefit. Aripiprazole was introduced which led to some improvement in behaviors, though an increase in stereotypic behaviors was noted. Sleep also became significantly disturbed with disinhibition noted.

Examination

When seen, he was unable to tolerate a stranger and seemed to become quite agitated. Later on, he was observed and seemed to demonstrate complex motor as well as vocal tics, stereotypic behaviors with poor attention, and overactivity. No seizures were noted. See Table 13.1.

Differential Diagnosis

The differential diagnoses at this stage included an undiagnosed developmental disorder such as attention deficit hyperactivity disorder (ADHD) and Tourette's syndrome (TS), an undiagnosed physical health condition, an underlying psychiatric

Table 13.1 Features which may help to discriminate tics from motor stereotypies

	Stereotypies	Motor tics
Age of onset	Earlier age of onset usually before the age of 3	Average age of onset of 5–7 years
Semiology	Consistent and fixed in pattern	Tend to evolve over time
Body area affected	Frequently involve the arms, hands, or entire body	Commonly seen in the eyes, face, head, and shoulders
Duration	Are more rhythmic and prolonged in duration	Usually involves brief contraction of muscle groups
Effect of distraction	Stop and cease	Can decrease tics

disorder such as bipolar disorder, and a seizure disorder or behavioral disturbances due to the underlying autism and intellectual disability.

Investigations

Behavioral monitoring was instituted and further developmental history was sought. Video recordings about behavioral problems were carried out. Precise documentation of behaviors with behavioral analysis was done. An MRI was considered but not done due to persistent challenging behaviors, and on balance it was felt that the risks of proceeding were too great. An EEG was considered not tolerable.

Progress

Video recordings demonstrated stereotypic behaviors, some of which were initially considered to be possible "seizures." Complex motor tics, vocal tics, and sensory perception behaviors were also noted on video recordings. Overactivity and impulsive behaviors were noted as well as restlessness and an inability to maintain concentration on any task.

The challenging behavior was considered to be of such a degree that intervention was necessary. Drug-to-drug interactions and possible drug toxicity were also considered possibilities. It was agreed with the family and carers to rationalize DM's medications.

Working diagnoses of ADHD and tic disorder were made. Carbamazepine was withdrawn gradually over subsequent months. Risperidone was gradually reduced to a dose of 1 mg a day. It was decided to treat empirically and atomoxetine was commenced and built up gradually to a dose of 50 mg a day. This led to significant improvement in DM's mental state with reduction in hyperactive and impulsive behaviors and improved attention. However the effects were not long lasting with an increase in agitation noted a few weeks after being on atomoxetine. A reduction in atomoxetine did not lead to any significant benefit. Medication sensitivity was considered to be one of the options.

It was decided to make further reductions in psychotropic medications. Sodium valproate, aripiprazole, and quetiapine were withdrawn completely over a 6–12 month period with regular behavioral interventions and monitoring. Ecological strategies were also instituted.

Further improvements in mental state were noted. DM became significantly more settled with a less aggression, hyperactivity, impulsivity, and agitation. His mood was more stable and he was able to enjoy and partake in leisure activities. His concentration was better and he was able to communicate and make his needs known. He continues to experience vocal and motor tics though these are more manageable.

He currently remains on risperidone 0.5 mg a day as the only psychotropic medication and has been on this for the last 12 months.

Diagnosis

The final diagnosis was of a tic disorder – Tourette's syndrome in someone with autism and intellectual disability.

What Did I Learn from This Case?

I learned a number of important lessons from this case.

Diagnosis was an important factor in this case, as it would inform prescribing. I found that differentiating different behavioral syndromes in people with autism could be challenging. Tics could resemble stereotypic behaviors, and emotional symptoms may suggest disorders such as ADHD or cyclical mood disorders such as bipolar disorder. ADHD was considered to be more of an appropriate diagnosis as opposed to bipolar disorder. Distinguishing ADHD and bipolar disorder can be challenging as features of distractibility, hyperactivity, impulsivity, and impaired attention and concentration are common to both disorders. However, this patient probably did not have any of these conditions as his response to medications demonstrated.

At times, some of the routine investigations open to people without intellectual disability cannot be incorporated in the management of people with intellectual disability, and the basic skills of history taking and observations are important. A good developmental history is important as in this case; it put the diagnosis of bipolar disorder to question.

This case highlights the role of drug prescribing in worsening clinical situations. Drug interaction and sensitivity seemed to play an important role in some of the behavioral problems this patient presented with. While as doctors we are sometimes required to "do something" and add or increase medication, when someone presents with behavioral problems, it is important to consider that some of the prescribing may contribute to agitation and restlessness and a gradual reduction in poly-prescribing can actually be helpful and improve overall quality of life as this case has shown.

Bibliography

Aman M, DeSmedt G, Derivan A, et al. Risperidone treatment of children with disruptive behaviour disorders and subaverage IQ: a double-blind, placebo-controlled study. Am J Psychiatry. 2002;159:1337–46.

Bodfish JW, Symons FJ, Parker DE, et al. Varieties of repetitive behaviour in autism: comparisons to mental retardation. J Autism Dev Disord. 2000;30:237–43.

Deb S, Clarke D, Unwin G. Using medication to manage behaviour problems among adults with a learning disability. Royal College of Psychiatrists Quick Reference Guide. 2006.

Chapter 14
Twitches and Fidgets Might Not Tell the Whole Story

Mary May Robertson, Valsamma Eapen, and Renata Rizzo

Case “A” was referred to our clinic and was seen by two authors (RR and MMR) first at the age of 6 years. His parents, Mr and Mrs X, described a history of abnormal movements since the age of 3 years; these included blinking and strange head movements.

Background History

His family was notable for a strong positive family history of Huntington’s disease (HD) on the paternal side. The father is a twin and one of eight siblings. Specifically, two of his sisters, one brother, and his mother had been diagnosed as having HD. A’s father did not attend the first two appointments, but A’s mother reported that the father was well but had chosen not to be tested for HD. The mother is one of seven

M.M. Robertson, MB, MD, DSc, FRCPCH, FRCP, FRCPsych (✉)
Emeritus (University College London), London, UK

Honorary University Cape Town, Cape Town, South Africa

St Georges Hospital, London, UK
e-mail: m.robertson@ucl.ac.uk

V. Eapen, MBBS, PhD, FRCPsych, FRANZCP
Academic Unit of Child Psychiatry South West Sydney (AUCS), School of Psychiatry, Mental Health Centre, Liverpool Hospital, University of New South Wales and Liverpool Hospital, Sydney, NSW, Australia
e-mail: v.eapen@unsw.edu.au

R. Rizzo, MD, PhD
Department of Medical and Pediatric Science, Azienda Policlinico-OVE, Catania University, Catania, Italy
e-mail: rerizzo@unict.it

J. Priller, H. Rickards (eds.), *Neuropsychiatry Case Studies*,
DOI 10.1007/978-3-319-42190-2_14

siblings with no known relevant family history. However when we interviewed her, we noted that she had some motor tics, to which she admitted having from time to time and, on direct questioning, also admitted that one of her sisters also had some "motor tics" but she could not be more specific. The mother had had a previous marriage resulting in two healthy children, a male and female aged 25 and 19 years, respectively.

After Mrs X married Mr X, she became pregnant three times, but miscarried on each occasion. At the age of 34 years, Mrs X conceived. The pregnancy was complicated by threatened miscarriage at around 4 months. At 40 weeks of gestation, she had an emergency cesarean section because the placenta actually broke. A baby boy, "A," was born, weighing 2,350 g, and his length was 49 cm. There was no jaundice. The first steps of psychomotor development were normal. He walked and began to talk at around 12 months. At the age of 3, he began nursery school without any problems. He then began to manifest movements that had the characteristics of "tics." From the age of 3–6, he continued to have "tics" which changed in nature but never disappeared. At the age of 6, he began his first year of primary school with good school performance. However the teacher apparently had complained that "A" roamed around the classroom inappropriately. Otherwise he was a well-behaved child. He made friends at school and had good relationships with them. "A" and his parents have always enjoyed a good relationship.

Examination and Investigations

Examination of "A" revealed a delightful child who interacted well and was cooperative. He reacted well to the environment; his talk was logical, relevant, and coherent; and he exhibited both motor and vocal tics. The motor tics we observed at interview included blinking, frowning, eyebrow raising, head nodding, head tilting backwards, head touching the shoulder, shoulder shrugging, as well as repetitive throat clearing. There was no evidence of depression, psychosis, or cognitive decline. After his first visit, we therefore clinically suspected Gilles de la Tourette syndrome (GTS), but in view of the very strongly positive paternal family history decided that we had to undertake specific investigations including DNA analysis for HD, ceruloplasmin, a brain MRI, and a Wechsler Intelligence Scale for Children-Revised (WISC-R). We arranged to see him after the investigations had been performed. All the investigations as detailed above were normal and he was negative for HD.

Progress

A was seen again for the second time, accompanied by both his parents at our specific request, and the family was assessed using the standardized schedules: the National Hospital Interview Schedule (NHIS) [1], the Diagnostic Confidence Index

(DCI) [2], the Yale Global Tic Severity Rating Scale (YGTSS) [3], and the Motor tic, Obsessions and compulsions, Vocal tic Evaluation Survey (MOVES) [4]. Family history revealed that on the maternal side, the mother, Mrs X, aged 42 years, had experienced both multiple motor and vocal tics since the age of 8 years, and she also had obsessions with both counting and cleaning. She had six siblings, four sisters, and two brothers. One of her sisters had severe depression with attempted suicide at the age of 15 years. Another sister also had severe depression with an attempted suicide and also a "religious obsession." Another of Mrs X's sisters had a son with severe ADHD, requiring special teaching, who had to be treated with medication. Yet another of her sisters had motor and vocal tics, a cleaning obsession, and hyperactivity. Finally the son of one brother had motor tics and a stutter.

Importantly, on the paternal side, the grandmother had confirmed HD and died at 55 years. The father Mr X had seven siblings. Two sisters and a brother had confirmed HD. A sister had severe depression. The diagnoses of the two of the five children of one of the sisters with HD included depression and chronic motor tics. One child aged 19 of the affected brother decided to have the HD test and was negative.

Examination and Further Investigations

"A" had a history of 25 motor tics (both simple and complex) and at least 5 vocal tics. His mother reported when questioned directly that he also had echolalia and echopraxia, but no coprolalia and palilalia nor palipraxia. In addition he had a particular song going over and over in his mind for no apparent reason. On history there was no evidence of obsessive-compulsive disorder (OCD), attention deficit hyperactivity disorder (ADHD), conduct disorder (CD), or rage attacks. He, however, had a counting obsession (arithmomania) in that he counted cars, children, and scooters, and we diagnosed this as OCB. He also had frequent nightmares and night terrors and had a spider phobia. On the YGTSS he scored 27 %, on the MOVES he scored 4/60, and on the DCI he scored 69 % (the tertiary clinic average for the DCI is 60 %) suggesting a diagnosis of GTS of mild to moderate severity.

During the interview, A's mother, Mrs X, was observed to exhibit blinking, winking, platysma tightening, eyebrow raising, a nasal twitch, and possible throat clearing. She then admitted to throat clearing as a child. We saw no abnormal movements in A's father, Mr X.

Differential Diagnosis

The obvious differential diagnosis was HD because of the positive family history. However the early age of onset of having involuntary movements from the age of 3 characterized by multiple motor and vocal tics suggested that this was a case of

GTS. Although there was a known strong positive paternal family history of HD, further detailed evaluation also revealed both motor and vocal tics in the mother and family history suggestive of GTS on the maternal side of the family. Further investigations found that he was negative for HD on genetic testing and there were no other abnormalities on any of the other investigations.

Diagnosis

Although initially when seen by RR at the age of 6, a diagnosis of GTS was suspected based on the clinical presentation that the motor and vocal tics had a waxing and waning course with one type of tic being replaced by another, which are all characteristic of Tourette syndrome, considering HD on the paternal side of the family, it was suggested that a diagnosis of HD had to be excluded. However, the father having had years of experience of devastating impact of HD on his side of the family took a very fatalistic view and had chosen for himself not to be tested for HD. The mother on the other hand considering that HD affected a number of female members of her husband's family wanted her son to take the test as she had a more optimistic view about the risks and its implications. He therefore underwent all laboratory tests including HD investigations even though predictive testing for less than 18 years is not normally done. The results were negative and he was then seen by RR and MMR and a diagnosis of GTS was confirmed. It is to be noted that in addition to the motor and vocal tics, he also exhibited tic-related behaviors such as echolalia and echopraxia and OCB in the form of arithmomania. The strong positive family history of GTS in the mother and other members of the maternal side of the family further supported this diagnosis.

What Did We Learn from This Case?

To the best of our knowledge, this case is one of the few in the literature to report a young patient with strong family history of both GTS and HD, thereby presenting significant diagnostic challenges. Moreover our case illustrates the ethical and clinical dilemma with regard to genetic testing when young patients present with involuntary movements and a positive family history of HD. This is particularly the case when complex tic symptoms are mistaken for HD symptoms or vice versa and in either scenario difficulties may ensue, which could lead to misdiagnosis.

The generally accepted diagnostic criteria for Gilles de la Tourette syndrome (GTS), Tourette syndrome, or Tourette's disorder include multiple motor tics and one or more vocal tics, lasting longer than a year (American Psychiatric Association (APA) [5]; World Health Organization (WHO) [6]). The age at onset of TS ranges from 2 to 21 years, with a mean of 7 years, while the onset of vocal tics is, later, usually around 11 years of age. Tics can be simple (e.g., eye blinking, nose twitching) or complex (e.g., squatting) [7]. Premonitory sensations are common. Simple vocalizations include sniffing, throat clearing, and coughing. Complex vocal or phonic tics include barking and the uttering of strings of words. Other features include echolalia (copying what others say), echopraxia (copying what others do), and palilalia (repeating the last word or part of sentence uttered by the individual). Coprolalia (inappropriate, involuntary, swearing) is uncommon, occurring in only 10–15 % of patients, usually starting at around 15 years, and another common and often disabling symptom of GTS is nonobscene socially inappropriate (NOSI) behaviors (for review see Robertson and Eapen [8]. Boys are more commonly affected, with the male and female ratio being 3:1. GTS was once considered to be uncommon, but no less than seven recent studies have remarkably consistent findings and suggest a prevalence of between 0.4 % and 1.76 % for youngsters aged 5–18 years. It was initially thought that GTS is a lifelong disorder, but Leckman et al. [9] have suggested that the prognosis is, in fact, better than previously thought and that the majority of symptoms disappeared in half of the patients by the age of 18 years. Further, adult-onset tic disorder has been described in the literature. In this regard, "tardive tourettism" after prolonged use of antipsychotics (neuroleptics) has been described [10], and Eapen et al. [11] reported adult-onset acquired tic disorder [12] following toxic exposure, vascular events, or other medical causes that constitute secondary tourettism. Cases of tardive and emergent chorea have also been described in patients with GTS [13]. Also, Lees et al. [14] reported a cohort of patients with GTS, in whom chorea was observed in two previously untreated patients.

While there are case reports in the literature where co-occurrence of GTS and HD symptoms has been described, the notable exception with our cases is the absence of family history of both conditions in the previous reports. The first case of childhood-onset TS, before the age of 10 years, and adult-onset HD was reported by Kerbeshian et al. [15] who described a 40-year-old man, ET, who had had GTS since childhood and later developed HD at about 26 years of age. Another case was reported by Jankovic and Ashizawa [16] of a man who at about the age of 31 years became depressed and had continuous irregular movements of his feet and restlessness in his legs. Some 8–10 years later, he began sniffing, having a "hacking" cough, having facial grimacing, jerking of his head, and other jerk-like movements. He frequently "choked" on drinks. He showed deterioration and his MMSE score was 20/30. DNA analysis confirmed HD mutation containing 47 CAG repeats. Family history revealed that on the paternal side, seven individuals had abnormal movements. The patient's mother was neurologically well. One brother had a "hacking cough" and other involuntary vocalizations, while a sister had some restlessness when she tried to fall asleep. The authors commented that their case illustrated the broad range of clinical manifestations of HD. We wonder whether or not the patient's 43-year-old brother had vocalizations only (i.e., part of the GTS spectrum) or also unusual signs of HD. Angelini et al. [17] described a child affected by HD who had signs and neurological features of "tourettism." The absence of family history and persisting normal MRI scans delayed the diagnosis of HD. An MRI scan 26 months after disease onset revealed bilateral atrophy in the putamen, and the diagnosis of HD was confirmed by genetic analysis. Alonso et al. [18] reported a 30-year-old male patient with HD, also confirmed by genetic studies (46 repeats of CAG triplets), who had presented with features of GTS, including multiple motors tics since his teenage years as well as vocal tics, bruxism, and self-injurious behavior with a compulsive element to it. The only relevant family history was that his paternal grandfather had "abnormal repetitive movements of the upper limbs" of adult onset. The patient's father was asymptomatic but showed 40 CAG repeats: it had not been possible to study the paternal grandfather.

Further, co-occurrence of other mental health and behavioral difficulties is common in both GTS and HD. In GTS, close to 90 % of clinic patients are observed to have ADHD (attention deficit hyperactivity disorder), OCB (obsessive-compulsive behavior), and OCD (obsessive-compulsive disorder), and when TS is associated with such related behaviors, the term "TS-Plus" is used [19]. In the case of HD, particularly in younger patients, mental and emotional symptoms have been described [20]. For example, repetitive and compulsive behaviors have been reported in both GTS [21] and HD [22], although perseveration is more common in HD and OCD in GTS. In a large multiply affected HD pedigree consisting of 31 members of two filial generations of whom 13 members showed symptoms of the disease, tic-like hyperkinesias and compulsive behaviors were encountered in some individuals [23]. Further, De Marchi et al. [24] reported individuals from a large HD pedigree with a high prevalence of OCD, two of whom responded to fluoxetine.

The diagnosis of HD can sometimes be challenging when there is no family history. Siesling et al. [25] studied 172 patients suspected of having Huntington's disease, and the family history was compared with the CAG repeat length and the clinical features to determine the extent to which CAG repeat length has allowed the diagnoses of additional patients, with atypical psychiatric or neurological disease, or those without a family history. Of the 172 patients, 126 had an expanded repeat, and of these, 77 had a positive, 8 a negative, 40 a suspect, and 1 an unknown family history. Of the 44 patients with a normal repeat length, four had a positive family history. Of the two patients with an intermediate repeat (between 30 and 36 repeats), one with a negative family history received a clinical diagnosis of GTS. Thus, in cases of HD where there is no family history or a positive genetic finding, diagnostic determination and differential diagnosis with other involuntary movement disorders can be challenging based on clinical information alone. In this regard, Muller et al. [26] described intrafamilial heterogeneity of facial hyperkinesias and considered whether or not the association of tics, cranial dystonia, and HD was by chance or not. Hebebrand et al. [27], however, reported that there was no association between the length of the (CAG) repeat of the HD gene and GTS.

Clinically, HD always follows a progressive course, even in youngsters [20]. This is in sharp contrast to GTS, which has a waxing and waning course and improves with age with majority of patients reporting that they become relatively tic-free by young adulthood [28]. Although tics typically have a younger age of onset during the developmental period, several cases of young-onset HD have been reported. One of the youngest childhood-onset suspected cases documented was in an infant aged 20 months who had a severe behavior disorder and who then died at 20 months. The case was unusual in that there was no documented family history, but the CT scan and neuropathology, particularly of the basal ganglia, were compatible with HD [29]. A girl of 12 years old with HD has also been reported [30]. Papapetropoulos et al. [31] also reported a very young case of HD who was a maternally transmitted case of HD with a very large trinucleotide repeat.

Further, the diagnostic criteria for GTS as per DSM-5 [5] include that the tic symptom is not attributable to the physiological effects of a substance (e.g., cocaine) or other medical conditions (e.g., Huntington's disease, post-viral encephalitis), which makes the diagnostic overlap between GTS and HD extremely challenging. In order to ascertain that the tic symptoms are not due to HD, it will be critical to trace the temporal sequence of the onset of tic symptoms. Given that the GTS has a mean age of onset of 6–7 years, it would often be the case that the tic symptoms predate any HD symptoms. While the presence of family history of both GTS and HD on the one hand can be confusing, it can also provide a certain degree of diagnostic confidence especially if the HD is on the paternal side of the family as it has been suggested that when the onset is in childhood, the affected child is about four times as likely to have inherited HD from the father than the mother [20]. However, the dilemma of making a clinical decision as to whether to do the genetic testing for HD in a young patient presenting with tic symptoms in the context of a family history of HD would require careful ethical considerations.

References

1. Robertson MM, Eapen V. The national hospital interview schedule for the assessment of Gilles de la Tourette syndrome and related behaviours. Int J Methods Psychiatr Res. 1996;6(4): 203–26.
2. Robertson MM, Banerjee S, Kurlan R, Cohen DJ, Leckman JF, McMahon W, Pauls DL, Sandor P, van de Wetering BJ. The Tourette syndrome diagnostic confidence index: development and clinical associations. Neurology. 1999;53(9):2108–12.
3. Leckman JF, Riddle MA, Hardin MT, Ort SI, Swartz KL, Stevenson J, Cohen DJ. The yale global tic severity scale: initial testing of a clinician-rated scale of tic severity. J Am Acad Child Adolesc Psychiatry. 1989;28(4):566–73.
4. Gaffney GR, Sieg K, Hellings J. The MOVES: a self-rating scale for Tourette's syndrome. J Child Adolesc Psychopharmacol. 1994;4(4):269–80.
5. American Psychiatric Association. Diagnostic and statistical manual of mental disorders – fifth edition (DSM-5). Washington, DC: American Psychiatric Publishing; 2013.
6. World Health Organisation. International classification of diseases and health related problems – tenth revision. Geneva: World Health Organisation; 1992.
7. Eapen V, McPherson S, Sneddon C, Crncec R. Tic disorders and learning disability: clinical characteristics, cognitive performance and co-morbidity. Australas J Spec Educ. 2013;37: 162–72.
8. Robertson MM, Eapen V. Whither the relationship between etiology and phenotype in Tourette syndrome. In: Martine D, Leckman JF, editors. Tourette syndrome. Oxford: Oxford University Press; 2013. p. 361–94.
9. Leckman JF, Zhang H, Vitale A, Lahnin F, Lynch K, Bondi C, Kim YS, Peterson BS. Course of tic severity in Tourette syndrome: the first two decades. Pediatrics. 1998;102(1 Pt 1):14–9.
10. Stahl SM. Tardive Tourette syndrome in an autistic patient after long-term neuroleptic administration. Am J Psychiatry. 1980;137(10):1267–9.

11. Fountoulakis KN, Samara M, Siapera M, Iacovides A. Tardive Tourette-like syndrome: a systematic review. Int Clin Psychopharmacol. 2011;26(5):237–42.
12. Eapen V, Lees AJ, Lakke JPWF, Trimble MR, Robertson MM. Adult onset tic disorders. Mov Disord. 2002;17(4):735–40.
13. Kompoliti K, Goetz CG. Hyperkinetic movement disorders misdiagnosed as tics in Gilles de la Tourette syndrome. Mov Disord. 1998;13(3):477–80.
14. Lees AJ, Robertson M, Trimble MR, Murray NM. A clinical study of gilles de la tourette syndrome in the United Kingdom. J Neurol Neurosurg Psychiatry. 1984;47(1):1–8.
15. Kerbeshian J, Burd L, Leech C, Rorabaugh A. Huntington disease and childhood-onset Tourette syndrome. Am J Med Genet. 1991;39(1):1–3.
16. Jankovic J, Ashizawa T. Tourettism associated with Huntington's disease. Mov Disord. 1995;10(1):103–5.
17. Angelini L, Sgrò V, Erba A, Merello S, Lanzi G, Nardocci N. Tourettism as clinical presentation of Huntington's disease with onset in childhood. Ital J Neurol Sci. 1998;19(6):383–5.
18. Alonso H1, Cubo-Delgado E, Mateos-Beato MP, Solera J, Gómez-Escalonilla CI, Jiménez-Jiménez FJ. Huntington's disease mimicking Tourette syndrome. Rev Neurol. 2004;39(10): 927–9.
19. Eapen V, Robertson MM. Are there distinct subtypes in Tourette Syndrome (TS)? Pure-TS versus TS-Plus and simple versus complex tics. Neuropsychiatr Dis Treat (Accepted 24 Sept 2014).
20. Gordon N. Huntington's disease of early onset or juvenile Huntington's disease. Hosp Med. 2003;64:576–80.
21. Eapen V, Robertson MM. Tourette syndrome and co-morbid obsessive compulsive disorder: therapeutic interventions. CNS Drugs. 2000;13(3):173–83.
22. Cummings JL, Cunningham K. Obsessive-compulsive disorder in Huntington's disease. Biol Psychiatry. 1992;31(3):263–70.
23. Gerstenbrand F, Klingler D. Phenomenology of Huntington chorea, analysis of a large family. Wien Klin Wochenschr. 1985;97(10):464–8.
24. De Marchi N1, Daniele F, Ragone MA. Fluoxetine in the treatment of Huntington's disease. Psychopharmacology (Berl). 2001;153(2):264–6.
25. Siesling S, M V-v de V, Losekoot M, Belfroid RD, Maat-Kievit JA, Kremer HP, Roos RA. Family history and DNA analysis in patients with suspected Huntington's disease. J Neurol Neurosurg Psychiatry. 2000;69(1):54–9.
26. Müller J, Wenning GK, Wissel J, Poewe W. Intrafamilial heterogeneity of facial hyperkinesias: chance association of tics, cranial dystonia, and Huntington's disease? Mov Disord. 2001;16(2):370–2.
27. Hebebrand J, Nöthen MM, Klug B, Wettke-Schäfer R, Camps A, Lisch S, Hemmer S, von Gontard A, Poustka F, Lehmkuhl G, et al. No association between length of the (CAG)n repeat of the Huntington's disease gene and Tourette's syndrome. Biol Psychiatry. 1995;37(3): 209–11.
28. Robertson MM, Eapen V. Tourette's: syndrome, disorder or spectrum? Classificatory challenges and an appraisal of the DSM criteria. Asian J Psychiatry. 2014 (in press).
29. Haslam RH, Curry B, Johns R. Infantile Huntington's disease. Can J Neurol Sci. 1983;10(3): 200–3.
30. Foldager S, Røijen SB. Early onset of Huntington disease. Ugeskr Laeger. 1996;158(17): 2398–9.
31. Papapetropoulos S, Lopez-Alberola R, Baumbach L, Russell A, Gonzalez MA, Bowen BC, Singer C. Case of maternally transmitted juvenile Huntington's disease with a very large trinucleotide repeat. Mov Disord. 2005;20(10):1380–3.

Chapter 15
Apathy in Huntington's Disease: Medicating the Patient, Spouse, Both, or None?

Harald Gelderblom

Motivated by his wife, BT comes to our Huntington's disease (HD) clinic. His wife deplores her husband's increasing inactivity and loss of interest during the preceding year. She reports that BT spends nearly all day lying on the couch, watching soaps or other programs without displaying any interest in what is shown. He used to take great interest in politics but stopped reading the newspaper or watching the news. Upon questioning, his wife deplores a lack of intimacy or other signs of interest in herself. Having been an active and animated person, BT is now in a constant state of friendly indifference without empathy or interest in family and friends. His daily routine needs organization and frequent prompting. Both spouses argue frequently, and her efforts at activating him are increasingly futile. The wife reports to see a psychiatrist for depression. BT himself does not understand his wife's complaints nor does he notice the sadness and desperation she expresses. He acknowledges, though, that he may not be as interested in his surroundings as he used to be, but considers this as age related. Also, he enjoys relaxing on the sofa, as he often feels tired during the day. He negates feeling sad, guilty, or hopeless, nor does he notice a feeling of low self-esteem. His wife confirms that she has not noticed any signs of depression.

Background History

Having been diagnosed with HD at the age of 54, BT has been consulting his neurologist regularly. He retired 3 years ago when motor symptoms became more obvious and bradyphrenia started to interfere with his demanding job as the head of the regional bureau of a lobby firm. At that time, citalopram was started due to a major

H. Gelderblom, MD
Abteilung Medizin, GKV-Spitzenverband, Berlin, Germany
e-mail: harald.gelderblom@gkv-spitzenverband.de

J. Priller, H. Rickards (eds.), *Neuropsychiatry Case Studies*,
DOI 10.1007/978-3-319-42190-2_15

depression with suicidal ideations. While chorea, and lately axial dystonia, slowly progressed, some symptomatic relief was achieved first with tiapride and recently with tetrabenazine. Motor symptoms started to have an impact on BT's daily functions. However, it was only his wife who perceived them as disturbing and stigmatizing. Recently, bradyphrenia became more obvious and BT developed perseverations. He constantly deplored low temperature within buildings and the need to wear several layers of clothes until he was sweating. The symptoms almost fully remitted under treatment with olanzapine (7.5 mg qd). At that time, problems with swallowing were infrequently noticed.

Examination

During the consultation, BT was cooperative but showed a lack of interest. He seemed unaffected by his personal situation as well as by the desperation of his wife. During the examination, he was unable to attend and maintain focus. At some point, he closed his eyes, which in turn provoked reproaches by his wife. On neurologic examination, a moderate bucco-oro-lingual chorea and chorea of all extremities was observed. In addition, BT showed predominantly axial dystonia, which interfered with positional stability. The UHDRS motor score was 28 points.

Progress

The patient's history as reported by his wife was indicative of apathy. A Structured Clinical Interview for Apathy in Dementia (SCIA-D) was performed and confirmed apathy. The 18 questions of the Apathy Evaluation Scale (AES) were answered by BT (AES-S for self), by his wife (AES-I for informant), and by the treating physician (AES-C for clinician), and a score of 38/54, 24/54, and 34/54 was calculated.

BT received four drugs for neuropsychiatric symptom management which all have the potential to induce or aggravate apathy, namely, citalopram, tetrabenazine, tiapride, and olanzapine. Their medical justification was considered and a tapering plan was formulated. Tapering of citalopram and olanzapine did not result in a reoccurrence of perseverations or symptoms of depression. BT did seem to be a bit more agile. Tapering of tetrabenazine resulted in a *reduction* of axial dystonia with a mild increase in chorea. The dysphagia remitted. His wife reported that the symptoms of apathy and bradyphrenia were also less severe. When tiapride was reduced below 150 mg tid, chorea significantly interfered with the motor skills necessary for daily function. The patient was then offered to participate in a crossover trial of bupropion 300 mg qd versus placebo for the treatment of apathy in HD. Shortly after the start of the study medication (initially placebo), his wife noticed a reduction of apathetic symptoms. BT allegedly made her compliments and finished some chores of daily routine. When meeting with friends, he stayed up longer. After crossover of study medication (change to bupropion), BT again became more apathetic but still more active than prior to study initiation. After the end of the study, bupropion was administered with less effect and an increase of apathetic symptoms during the following year.

Differential Diagnosis

BT came to the HD clinic with severe lack of motivation, initiative, and drive as well as emotional blunting suggestive of apathy, the most frequent psychiatric symptom in HD. Depression as the major differential diagnosis had to be excluded, which may be difficult, as symptoms overlap. In most cases, however, differentiation between apathy and depression is not challenging. Neither BT nor his wife reported signs of depression. During psychiatric evaluation, BT did not appear depressed. Pharmacologic induction or—more frequent—aggravation of apathy had to be considered. In HD symptom management, medications of concern are antipsychotics including tiapride, tetrabenazine, SSRIs, and benzodiazepines. Their effect on apathetic symptoms, however, varies significantly. Often tapering of these drugs is indicated. In BT's case, after tapering of olanzapine and citalopram, neither perseverations nor symptoms of depression reappeared. Tapering of tetrabenazine led to a marked reduction of symptoms of apathy, axial rigidity, dysphagia, and bradyphrenia. Chorea, however, was aggravated. When tiapride was reduced to 400 mg qd, chorea interfered with fine motor skills, so that the daily dosage had to be raised to 500 mg qd.

Diagnosis

A clinical diagnosis of apathy was made, supported by the SCIA-D. The AES helped to evaluate the severity of symptoms and supported the clinical impression of BT's lack of insight. Aggravation of apathetic symptoms by psychotropic medication became obvious once tapering was initiated.

What Did I Learn from This Case?

The present case reveals some characteristic features of apathy in HD. I learned that it is helpful to consider the following aspects when treating HD patients with apathy: (1) Always *ask* for the symptoms of apathy, since apathy is common in HD, especially in the more advanced stages of the disease. However, patients do not report symptoms of apathy *because they are apathetic*. (2) Do ask the informant, as insight of the patient decreases, whereas apathy increases with disease progression.

Keep in mind that informants may not notice apathetic symptoms, as they evolve slowly during the course of the disease. (3) Take into account the circumstances, personality, and health status of the caretaker, as these factors may influence the dynamics between the patient and caretaker and the latter's weighing of apathetic symptoms. Your judgment may well differ from those of the patient and the caretaker and improves the more you focus on apathy during your care for patients with neurodegenerative diseases. (4) Nearly all drugs prescribed for the symptomatic treatment in HD may induce or—more often—aggravate apathy. As neuropsychiatric symptoms change over the course of the disease, tapering is often justified. (5) After stopping or reducing medications that may induce apathy in HD patients, determine a baseline of apathetic symptoms using an instrument like the AES. (6) When you intend to start the patient on a medication to lessen apathy, be aware that there is no available clinical evidence. One result of our crossover trial was a treatment, not a drug effect. This observation supports my experience that it is participation and activation—difficult as it may be—and the development of a perspective for both, patient and caretaker, that may still be the best therapy for apathy.

Bibliography

Krishnamoorthy A, Craufurd D. Treatment of apathy in Huntington's disease and other movement disorders. Curr Treat Options Neurol. 2011;13:508–19.

Levy R, Dubois B. Apathy and the functional anatomy of the prefrontal cortex-basal ganglia circuits. Cereb Cortex. 2006;16:916–28.

Starkstein SE, Leentjens AF. The nosological position of apathy in clinical practice. J Neurol Neurosurg Psychiatry. 2008;79:1088–92.

van Duijn E, Giltay EJ, Zitman FG, Roos RAC, van der Mast RC. Measurement of psychopathology in Huntington's disease, the critical role of caregivers. J Nerv Ment Dis. 2010a;198: 329–33.

van Duijn E, Reedeker N, Giltay EJ, Roos RA, van der Mast RC. Correlates of apathy in Huntington's disease. J Neuropsychiatr Clin Neurosci. 2010b;22:287–94.

Part III
Functional Disorders

Chapter 16
Diagnostic Layers

Tiago Teodoro and Mark J. Edwards

This 44-year-old, right-handed lady was well until 5 years before attending our clinic, when she tripped and fell down a flight of stairs. She developed an acute left-sided hemifacial droop and leg weakness. Examination showed a positive left Hoover's sign (the power of left hip extension was zero when tested directly, but was normal when triggered by right hip flexion). She had a cranial CT scan, cranial and spine MRI, and multimodal evoked potentials, which were normal. She was given the diagnosis of a functional neurological disorder and started on treatment with fluoxetine and diazepam.

Her condition progressively worsened, especially in the 2 years prior to being seen in our clinic. She had persistent left-sided weakness and developed left arm tremor and arm pain, slowness of movements, and walking difficulties. She described blocking or freezing of gait when she was out in public and ended up walking with a stick indoors and using a wheelchair outside.

Nine months before attending to our clinic, she had had a very severe symptom exacerbation, coinciding with a urinary tract infection. This improved back to her previous baseline with physiotherapy in a neurological rehabilitation unit.

T. Teodoro, MD
Department of Cardiovascular and Cell Sciences, St George's University of London, London, UK

Department of Neurosciences, Hospital de Santa Maria, Lisbon, Portugal

Instituto de Medicina Molecular, Lisbon, Portugal
e-mail: tteodoro@sgul.ac.uk

M.J. Edwards, PhD (✉)
Institute of Cardiovascular and Cell Sciences, St. George's University of London, London, UK
e-mail: medwards@sgul.ac.uk

J. Priller, H. Rickards (eds.), *Neuropsychiatry Case Studies*,
DOI 10.1007/978-3-319-42190-2_16

Examination

She had marked facial hypomimia, reduced blink rate, and normal eye movements. The left side of her body was stiff and had a tremor that was possible to distract to some extent but not completely. Repetitive movements were slow, although not typically bradykinetic. She had difficulty in recruiting muscle power in the left leg, but it was possible to make this power normalize by getting her to flex her right hip (positive Hoover's sign). Gait was slow and unsteady.

Diagnostic Formulation

1. *Functional movement disorder* (*FMD*) – accounting for the initial presentation with focal neurological deficits and positive physical signs of functional weakness and also for some of the present deficits
2. *Parkinson's disease* – contributing to her progressive worsening, with hypokinetic features and gait impairment with description of gait freezing

Investigations

- DAT-SPECT scan: asymmetric (R>L) striatal presynaptic dopaminergic deficit

Final Diagnosis

1. *Parkinson's disease*
2. *FMD*

Management and Progress

1. *Parkinson's disease*: she was started on ropinirole which was well tolerated and produced significant clinical improvement.
2. *FMD*: *patient education* – functional symptoms were explained as real, having distinguishing characteristics and not being "imagined," "put on," or "all in the mind." Risk factors for the development of FMD were discussed including the role of physical injury and psychological stress. Physiotherapy-based treatment was deemed most appropriate for her in the absence of significant psychopathology, but this was postponed to determine the beneficial effect of treatment of the Parkinson's disease and education about FMD.

What Did I Learn from This Case?

Our patient had a sudden onset of FMD following a physical injury, with subsequent development of Parkinson's disease (PD) in parallel with the functional symptoms.

The diagnosis of FMD can be made with reasonable confidence on the basis of positive features of the history and examination. When made in this fashion, the diagnosis is stable over time, and there is rarely another explanation found for the original symptoms at long-term follow-up [1]. However, patients with FMD may well have other medical problems or can develop other medical problems over time. Sometimes the presence of the FMD can cloud the adequate assessment and management of these problems. This is particularly the case if the diagnosis of FMD produces alienation of the patient from medical services and if reassessment of new/progressive symptoms is blocked. This block can happen either because the patient has lost trust in health professionals or if health professionals are frightened of triggering another round of "organic" investigations which they feel will exacerbate the FMD. This is a complex issue, but in this case, new symptoms had developed over time and a simple clinical reevaluation by neurology was reasonable to determine the need for further investigations and a reevaluation of the diagnosis. Most of the time, this would confirm that the only diagnosis is the original one, but sometimes, as in this case, an additional diagnosis is made. It has also been our experience that the presence of FMD can prevent adequate treatment of comorbid problems, for example, chronic migraine, which when treated successfully can produce improvement in quality of life for the patient. *The first teaching point of our case is therefore that comorbidity occurs in patients with FMD and that comorbid problems should be treated as they would normally. Clinical reevaluation is reasonable in the situation of new or progressive symptoms and when handled correctly should not lead to exacerbation of the functional symptoms.*

The second teaching point that this case illustrates is the common precipitation of FMD by physical events. In one retrospective study, physical events preceded the onset of a functional movement disorder in 80 % of patients, with injury and infection being the most common triggers [2]. Our patient developed the initial symptoms after falling down a flight of stairs. Interestingly, 38 % of a cohort of functional movement disorder patients fulfilled criteria for the diagnosis of a panic attack during their physical "trigger" event [2]. Physical events generate unusual sensory data that may be abnormally processed and constitute a substrate for the generation of abnormal movements [2]. An accompanying panic attack may increase the salience of those unusual sensations or generate additional physical symptoms such as tremor [2].

A third teaching point that this case highlights is the unexpectedly high frequency of functional neurological symptoms in patients with PD. Epidemiological studies have reported that somatoform disorders are more frequent in PD and dementia with Lewy bodies (DLBs) in comparison with other neurodegenerative disorders [3, 4]. Functional movement disorders may either precede or follow PD diagnosis [5]. The most common FMD in PD appears to be functional tremor, followed by gait disorder and fixed dystonia [5]. The overlay of these disorders may confound diagnosis and management of either of them. Indeed, overlaying functional symptoms in PD may lead to significant disability and motivate therapy escalation, including seeking deep brain stimulation [5]. Therefore, functional symptoms should be always considered when managing unexpected clinical deteriorations or treatment-refractory symptoms in PD [5]. The presence of functional symptoms may predate the onset of PD, as in our case. We have suggested elsewhere [5] that there may be pathophysiological consequences of the neurodegenerative process that happens in PD, specifically the loss of habitual/automatic movement control, and the dependence on more conscious "attention-full" movement control [6] may predispose people with PD to developing functional movement disorders [5, 7].

References

1. Stone J, Smyth R, Carson A, Lewis S, Prescott R, Warlow C, et al. Systematic review of misdiagnosis of conversion symptoms and "hysteria". BMJ. 2005;331(7523):989.
2. Pareés I, Kojovic M, Pires C, Rubio-Agusti I, Saifee TA, Sadnicka A, et al. Physical precipitating factors in functional movement disorders. J Neurol Sci. 2014;338(1–2):174–7.
3. Onofrj M, Bonanni L, Manzoli L, Thomas A. Cohort study on somatoform disorders in Parkinson disease and dementia with Lewy bodies. Neurology. 2010;74(20):1598–606.
4. Onofrj M, Thomas A, Tiraboschi P, Wenning G, Gambi F, Sepede G, et al. Updates on somatoform disorders (SFMD) in Parkinson's disease and dementia with Lewy bodies and discussion of phenomenology. J Neurol Sci. 2011;310(1–2):166–71.
5. Pareés I, Saifee TA, Kojovic M, Kassavetis P, Rubio-Agusti I, Sadnicka A, et al. Functional (psychogenic) symptoms in Parkinson's disease. Mov Disord Off J Mov Disord Soc. 2013;28(12):1622–7.
6. Edwards MJ, Adams RA, Brown H, Pareés I, Friston KJ. A Bayesian account of "hysteria". Brain J Neurol. 2012;135(Pt 11):3495–512.
7. Redgrave P, Rodriguez M, Smith Y, Rodriguez-Oroz MC, Lehericy S, Bergman H, et al. Goal-directed and habitual control in the basal ganglia: implications for Parkinson's disease. Nat Rev Neurosci. 2010;11(11):760–72.

Chapter 17
A Case of a Familial "Dopamine-Responsive" Movement Disorder

J.M. Gelauff and M.A.J. de Koning-Tijssen

History

Patient A, a 46-year-old woman, was seen at the movement disorder outpatient clinic because of involuntary movements and postures and painful cramping for 1 year. The symptoms acutely started with cramps in her left leg during a bicycle ride. Over several weeks this gradually worsened toward gait problems, tiredness, and inward posturing of the left foot, intermittent tremor in the left hand, and jerky movements of the trunk. At the time of presentation, the posturing and fatigue were most prominent.

Background History

One year previously, the patient was hospitalized because of progressive left hemiparesis and tremor, at the time the diagnosis functional movement disorder was considered. There was no significant past medical history.

Examination and Investigations

Neurological examination showed a slow forward arm rolling test on the left side and inversion of the left foot when walking. In rest, no dystonia was observed. Tandem gait was abnormal. Jerks and tremor in the left arm were observed

J.M. Gelauff, MD (✉) • M.A.J. de Koning-Tijssen, MD, PhD
Department of Neurology, University Medical Center Groningen,
Groningen, The Netherlands
e-mail: j.m.gelauff@umcg.nl; M.A.J.de.Koning-Tijssen@umcg.nl

J. Priller, H. Rickards (eds.), *Neuropsychiatry Case Studies*,
DOI 10.1007/978-3-319-42190-2_17

intermittently during the examination and were distractible. There was a subjective hypesthesia of the left arm.

Polymyography showed a tremor that was variable in amplitude, intermittent, and distractible pointing toward a functional origin. A brain MRI did not show any abnormalities.

Diagnosis and Initial Treatment

Based on the history, neurological examination, and polymyography, the diagnosis functional movement disorder was made. The abrupt start of the symptoms and pain in the history, fixed posturing of the foot, distractibility of the tremor, and atypical gait disorder were instrumental for the diagnosis. The findings of variability and distractibility in the polymyography confirmed this. Physiotherapy was tried without any desirable effect. Therefore rehabilitation therapy was started.

Follow-Up

The patient was seen for further follow-up at the outpatient clinic and mentioned that her elderly sister suffered from the same complaints. Also her great grandmother was said to have had abnormal posturing of one hand and one leg.

Her sister (patient B) was seen for consultation. In her case, symptoms started with a fall in the supermarket 3.5 years ago. She developed painful cramping and posturing of the left arm and jerks in the left arm. Furthermore, she experienced progressive symptoms of tiredness and gait problems. At neurological examination her gait was wiggly, with inward posturing of the left foot and elevation of the left shoulder. She had altered fixed posturing and intermittent distractible jerks of the left arm, and the finger tapping was slow, with hesitations, without a decrease in amplitude. She was diagnosed in the past with a conversion disorder.

Management

Based on the dystonic posturing during walking and the positive family history with identical complaints in her sister and the history of the great grandmother, dopamine-responsive dystonia (DRD) was considered, although we still considered the diagnosis of a functional movement disorder as most likely. A dopamine trial was initiated in our index patient with a dose of 62.5 mg three times daily. Within a few days, there was a remarkable effect. Her gait improved and the abnormal movements, including the posturing, disappeared. Also the patient reported to be less tired and she could return to work.

Because dopamine had had such a good effect on patient A, her sister was also treated with dopamine (62.5 mg once daily), with good effect after 1.5 weeks. Posturing in the arm and walking improved; however pain and fatigue remained.

Differential Diagnosis

DRD was considered a reasonable explanation of the symptoms, because of the favorable response to dopamine treatment and the presumed familiarity. Dystonia, gait problems, and bradykinesia, which were all observed in our patients, are described in DRD.

However, there were also signs that indicated a possible functional origin. The tremor that accompanied the dystonic symptoms was variable in amplitude, intermittent, and distractible. Furthermore there was fatigue and pain, which often coexist with functional neurological symptoms. There was a fixed inversion of the foot, which is not an exclusive feature but definitely a common phenotype of functional dystonia. Another argument against the diagnosis of DRD was the age of onset in these sisters. Typically, symptoms of DRD start in childhood or adolescence, although older ages of onset have been reported in literature [1].

Follow-Up

After a few months, while waiting for the genetic results, symptoms deteriorated in both patients. The abnormal posturing, tiredness, and abnormal movements returned, as did the gait problems, despite an increase in dose of dopamine up to 93,75 mg three times daily.

Further Investigations

A DNA test was requested in both patients. The most frequent form of DRD is caused by a mutation in the guanosine triphosphate cyclohydrolase 1 (GCH1) gene, which is inherited autosomal dominantly [2]. In our cases, an autosomal dominant inheritance pattern with reduced penetrance could be present. However, no mutation was found in this gene (or in other dopamine-responsive dystonia genes). We also excluded a deletion by multiplex ligation-dependent probe amplification.

A lumbar puncture in patient B did not show abnormalities in the dopamine metabolism.

Final Diagnosis

The diagnosis of a functional movement disorder was based on clinical findings and examination. Dopamine-responsive dystonia was excluded based on the negative DNA tests, normal cerebral fluid, and recurrence of symptoms during dopamine treatment.

What Did I Learn from This Case?

As we have seen in this case, it can be difficult to distinguish DRD from a functional movement disorder. Although DRD is a rare disorder, it remains important to keep it in mind, as it is one of the few causes of dystonia that is highly treatable.

In general, functional gait disorders, which were prominent in our two patients, are considered the most difficult to diagnose of all functional motor symptoms. The distinction between DRD and functional dystonia is particularly difficult, as the main diagnostic finding in DRD is a rapid response to dopamine administration [3], while functional movement disorders are defined as movement disorders that respond to nonphysiological maneuvers, among which often a strong placebo response [4]. In functional dystonia, Edwards et al. showed a dramatic and very rapid response to botulinum toxin injections, which was attributed to a placebo effect [5]. One of the objections invoked in the ethical discussion on placebo use in the treatment of functional symptoms is that the response would often be short lasting. In our patients, the effect (partially) remained for several months, but indeed deteriorated eventually.

The familial aspect in this case was both confounding and interesting. As the sisters developed highly comparable symptoms at around the same age, this prompted us to think of DRD. However we learned from this case that a functional movement disorder can be familial as well, as has been described before [6].

References

1. Lee WW, Jeon BS. Clinical spectrum of dopa-responsive dystonia and related disorders. Curr Neurol Neurosci Rep. 2014;14(7):461.
2. Ichinose H, Ohye T, Takahashi E, Seki N, Hori T, Segawa M, Nomura Y, Endo K, Tanaka H, Tsuji S, Fujita K, Nagatsu T. Hereditary progressive dystonia with marked diurnal fluctuation caused by mutations in the GTP cyclohydrolase I gene. Nat Genet. 1994;8:236–42.
3. Nutt JG, Nygaard TG. Response to levodopa treatment in dopa-responsive dystonia. Arch Neurol. 2001;58(6):905.
4. Edwards MJ, Fotopoulou A, Pareés I. Neurobiology of functional (psychogenic) movement disorders. Curr Opin Neurol. 2013;26(4):442–7.
5. Edwards MJ, Bhatia KP, Cordivari C. Immediate response to botulinum toxin injections in patients with fixed dystonia. Mov Disord. 2011;26(5):917–8.
6. Stamelou M, Cossu G, Edwards MJ, Murgia D, Pareés I, Melis M, Bhatia KP. Familial psychogenic movement disorders. Mov Disord. 2013;28(9):1295–8.

Chapter 18
Facial Spasm Can Look Like Facial Weakness in Patients with Functional Disorders

Jon Stone

BL is a 42-year-old female businesswoman who presented to emergency services with a 6 h history of progressive unilateral sensory and motor disturbance in her face, arm, and leg. She had woken with some tingling on the right side of her face which she had put down to feeling tired. About 3 h later, her daughter aged 9 noticed that her face looked "funny." When the patient looked in the mirror, she saw that her mouth was drooping on the right-hand side. She also became aware at the same time of some weakness and numbness in her right arm, especially in her hand. Her husband was familiar with the FAST test (Face, Arm, Speech Test) for the community recognition of stroke, and they immediately phoned emergency services who took her to accident and emergency. There was no associated headache. She had no past relevant medical history.

Background History

She was an articulate, educated woman who admitted she had been working long hours on her business and was also having to deal with some difficult neighbors, but she didn't think she'd been particularly stressed. She had been a little tired recently, but there was no history of symptoms compatible either with depression or anxiety.

J. Stone, MB, ChB, FRCP, PhD
Department of Clinical Neurosciences, University of Edinburgh, Western General Hospital, Edinburgh, UK
e-mail: Jon.Stone@ed.ac.uk; jstone@skull.dcn.ed.ac.uk

J. Priller, H. Rickards (eds.), *Neuropsychiatry Case Studies*, DOI 10.1007/978-3-319-42190-2_18

Examination

On arrival she was reported by general medical staff to have right facial droop and weak right arm and leg (although the clinical examination was the first time she'd been aware of leg weakness as a problem). She was investigated with a normal MRI brain scan including diffusion-weighted imaging (DWI) which is sensitive to acute stroke. MRI brain was repeated at 5 days and remained normal. CT angiography of the great vessels, carotids, and vertebral arteries was also normal excluding dissection. ECG and echocardiogram were normal as were routine blood test including a thrombophilia screen. Around 1 week after admission, she was referred to neurology services.

Differential Diagnosis

At this stage, based on the information given, there is a wide differential diagnosis which includes some kind of pathology in the left cerebral hemisphere. Before the normal imaging, it would certainly be reasonable to consider the following among others:

- Stroke. Although the gradual onset and positive sensory symptoms ("tingling") should have already put you off this diagnosis.
- Migraine. Common things being common, migraine should be high up the list of diagnostic possibilities in someone with an evolving sensorimotor disturbance. She didn't have a headache although migrainous aura without headache does occur.
- Demyelination/inflammation. The tempo of onset would be OK for this, and she is at an age where she is at risk for a first presentation of multiple sclerosis or some other inflammatory disorders such as lupus, sarcoidosis, or vasculitis.
- Metabolic problem. Hypoglycemia and other metabolic problems can present as stroke mimics.

With a normal MRI scan and blood tests, the differential diagnosis becomes more restricted. A stroke causing face, arm *and* leg weakness is more or less ruled out by the normal DWI since this would have to be a stroke covering quite a large territory of the brain. Inflammation in the spinal cord can cause arm and leg weakness but not facial symptoms. Migraine is one of the few diagnoses still tenable.

Progress

At review by neurology, it was clear that although she superficially appeared to have a facial droop, in fact, the problem was caused by unilateral contraction of the platysma, and there was jaw deviation to the right. The problem was therefore one of muscle *overactivity*, not underactivity (Figs. 18.1 and 18.2), and so the previous differential diagnosis was no longer valid. Such an appearance is almost

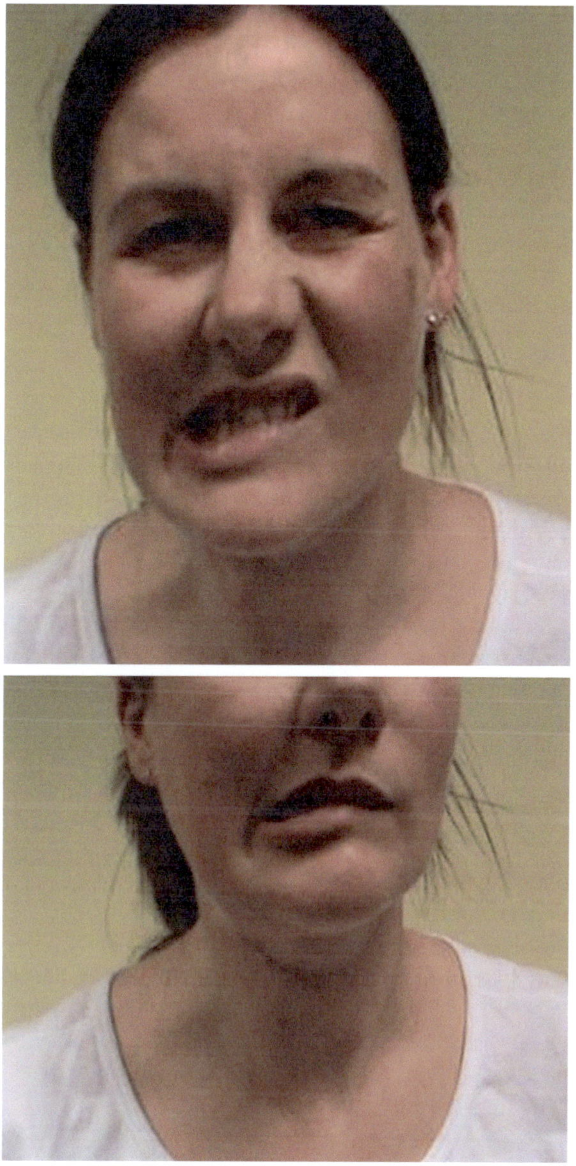

Figs. 18.1 and 18.2 Functional facial spasm with contraction of the platysma on the right and jaw deviation leading to a misleading appearance of lower facial "droop"

pathognomonic of functional facial spasm. This has been increasingly recognized in recent years although it was described extensively in the late nineteenth century also. In addition the weakness affecting her arm and leg had several qualities typical of functional limb weakness:

- She had a strongly positive Hoover's sign in the right leg (right hip extension was weak but returned to normal with contralateral hip flexion against resistance).
- She had a positive thigh abductor test (right hip abduction was weak but returned to normal with contralateral hip abduction against resistance).

- She had global weakness of all muscle groups in the arm and leg instead of a pyramidal/upper motor neuron pattern that you would expect from stroke or any other brain lesion. Pyramidal distribution weakness describes weakness of the extensor greater than the flexors in the arms and the "other way round" in the legs.
- She had dense sensory loss in the right hand, even to nail bed pressure, which occurs sometimes in functional disorders but rarely in neurological disease.
- The sensory loss was quite sharply demarcated and circumferential in a "long glove" distribution in the right hand.

Diagnosis

The diagnosis was functional neurological disorder (also described as conversion disorder, dissociative motor disorder, and psychogenic movement disorder), based on multiple positive features on the examination. In this case one could make an argument that the patient had been stressed, and while this was important to address in treatment, it would have been dangerous to base the diagnosis on this. In reality it is more likely that she did have some migrainous sensory disturbance in her face which had acted as a trigger for the rest of her symptoms. The understandable anxiety regarding a stroke, reinforced by the concern and diagnosis of stroke by hospital doctors, would have only amplified her symptoms.

Progress After Diagnosis

She responded well to a positive explanation of her diagnosis as a genuine functional disorder. She was shown all these signs with an emphasis on how they demonstrated the potential for reversibility of her symptoms. She found physiotherapy very helpful including a TENS machine to help her improve her sensory loss. At a later date, she realized that she had been "burning the candle at both ends" and that this had led her to be vulnerable to this episode although the triggering factor may have been migraine. She returned to work but with less hours and minimal residual symptoms about 6 months later.

Learning Points from This Case

This case illustrates the importance of not stereotyping patients with functional disorders. This diagnosis had not been entertained initially partly because the patient was articulate, educated, and "reasonable." It is important to be able to recognize functional facial spasm since it is actually one of the commoner functional presentations in neurology and has typical features, even though it has been neglected until recently. Her case also demonstrates the importance of making a diagnosis of a functional movement disorder, not on the basis of the personality of the patient, or even the presence or absence of life stress, but looking at the nature of the presenting symptoms and detecting positive findings on examination. Her recovery was led primarily by skilled physiotherapy, and it proved to be more useful to gain improvement in her movement symptoms first before exploring general vulnerabilities to her symptoms at a later date.

This patient described her story on BBC Radio 4 program "Inside Health." This is available to listen to in the UK as a podcast at http://downloads.bbc.co.uk/podcasts/radio4/medmatters/medmatters_20121009-2130a.mp3

Bibliography

Daum C, Hubschmid M, Aybek S. The value of "positive" clinical signs for weakness, sensory and gait disorders in conversion disorder: a systematic and narrative review. J Neurol Neurosurg Psychiatry. 2014;85:180–90.

Fasano A, Valadas A, Bhatia KP, Prashanth LK, Lang AE, Munhoz RP, et al. Psychogenic facial movement disorders: clinical features and associated conditions. Mov Disord. 2012;27:1544–51.

Kaski D, Bronstein AM, Edwards MJ, Stone J. Cranial functional (psychogenic) movement disorders. Lancet Neurol. 2015;14:1196–205.

Nielsen G, Stone J, Matthews A, Brown M, Sparkes C, Farmer R, et al. Physiotherapy for functional motor disorders: a consensus recommendation. J Neurol Neurosurg Psychiatry. 2015;86:1113–9.

Stone J, LaFrance WC, Brown R, Spiegel D, Levenson JL, Sharpe M, et al. Conversion disorder: current problems and potential solutions for DSM-5. J Psychosom Res. 2011;71:369–76.

Stone J. The bare essentials: functional symptoms in neurology. Pract Neurol. 2009;9:179–89.

Chapter 19
Review of Notes Documenting Initial Treatment Is Crucial in the Assessment of Acquired Brain Injury

Killian Welch

TR is a 20-year-old man who was admitted to a neurobehavioral rehabilitation unit due to concerns about cognitive impairment, irritability, and explosive anger episodes. He had experienced a head injury in an assault 2.5 years earlier. The family reported this had been associated with "water on the brain," he had been in hospital for several days, had briefly been in intensive care unit, and subsequently had significant memory problems. They showed a newspaper clipping of the patient with facial injuries and an airway in place. Psychiatric assessment 2 months after the injury recorded a score of 60 on the Addenbrooke's Cognitive Assessment Revised and also flashbacks and nightmares related to the assault, hypervigilance, avoidance, emotional blunting, and withdrawal from others. As symptoms did not improve with initial treatment, he had input from a community brain injury rehabilitation team and had already had a 4-month admission to a neurorehabilitation unit. Comprehensive cognitive assessment during this admission demonstrated substantial impairment in verbal and visual memory, executive function (planning, judgment, and task switching), working memory, and speed of processing. The admission ended in an unplanned manner due to aggression toward the staff.

Background History

The assault in which TR experienced his head injury involved being hit over the head with a hammer and stabbed in the chest and face with a broken bottle. TR reported remembering nothing of the assault other than an isolated memory of attempting to jump out of a window to escape. TR's family reported a normal

K. Welch, MBChB, MPhil, MD
Robert Fergusson Unit, Royal Edinburgh Hospital, Edinburgh, UK
e-mail: Killian.Welch@nhslothian.scot.nhs.uk

J. Priller, H. Rickards (eds.), *Neuropsychiatry Case Studies*,
DOI 10.1007/978-3-319-42190-2_19

developmental history, with average performance at school. They reported his personality had completely changed following the head injury, going from warm and easygoing to irritable and aggressive.

TR lived in a midsized, deprived town with a strong gang culture. His assailant was known to him and had been released from prison after serving 12 months of a 32-month sentence by the time of TR's admission. TR thought it likely he would be murdered, but denied fear of this saying he "had had a good life" and "if it happens, it happens."

Examination

TR presented as anxious and hypervigilant. He initially completely refused to leave the ward, even in the company of the staff. Formal testing of cognition again indicated impairment in various spheres, with amnestic deficits particularly pronounced. He frequently lost items, was unable to learn his way around the hospital, and after several weeks, had still not learned the names of any staff members. Speech and language assessment recorded a severe receptive and expressive dysphasia, and he required prompting with even basic tasks in occupational therapy assessment. Neurological examination was normal.

Investigations

Extensive blood investigations, MRI, and ECG were normal. SPECT scan revealed reduced cortical uptake in a patchy fashion, particularly within the frontal and parietal lobes (see Fig. 19.1).

Progress

Treatment initially focused on introduction of compensatory approaches for cognitive deficits (diaries, calendars, etc.), psychoeducation about anxiety/post-traumatic stress disorder (PTSD), training in relaxation/diaphragmatic breathing, and an exposure program initially focused on increasing time off the ward. Though pharmacological treatments for anxiety/PTSD had been trialled previously, compliance had been poor. He was treated with a combination of Sertraline and Trazodone, the latter particularly to assist with marked initial insomnia.

Within 2 months of admission, some inconsistencies in cognitive performance were observed by the nursing staff. For example, he was able to order a Chinese takeaway from a menu though language impairments remained severe on formal assessment, and he could reliably keep score during games of table tennis. By this time copies of medical notes relating to initial hospital treatment had also been obtained.

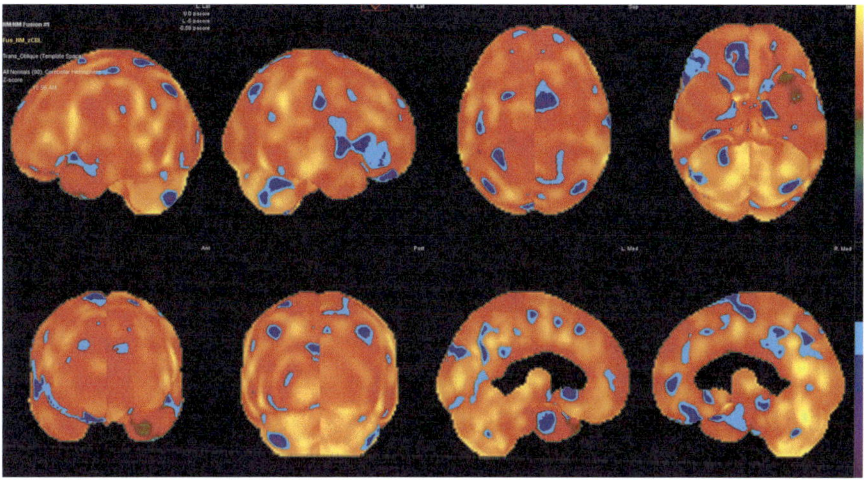

Fig. 19.1 Surface-shaded display derived from SPECT scan. *Blue-/purple*-shaded areas demonstrate perfusion well below the normal range. There is reduced relative uptake in a patchy fashion, but this is not indicative of any particular diagnosis. The images were acquired on a GE Discovery 670 gamma camera, and the surface-shaded display was generated on a MIMneuro workstation (Image provided by Nuclear Medicine, Western General Hospital, Edinburgh)

These recorded him GCS 12 (E3, V4, M5) at admission to hospital. Six hours later he was recorded as GCS 15. After surgical intervention for facial injuries and interview by the police, he was discharged, total duration of admission being 2 days.

Diagnosis

At the time of admission, it was assumed TR had severe cognitive impairment secondary to traumatic brain injury. He had already had an admission to a neurorehabilitation unit (during which no doubts about this diagnosis had, to our knowledge, been raised), and his presentation was initially indistinguishable from that of someone with a severe brain injury. Review of medical notes relating to the initial injury did not however seem consistent with the severity of impairment, suggesting impairment was either attributable to another brain pathology or was functional. Normal bloods, EEG, and structural imaging suggested the latter, and as time went on and inconsistencies in presentation emerged, confidence in this diagnosis increased.

Progress After Diagnosis

TR's cognitive difficulties were positively reframed as attributable to abnormalities in the brain function rather than structure and consequently potentially reversible. Reassuring test findings were discussed with him, and a formulation collaboratively developed emphasizing how impaired attention and concentration developing in the context of PTSD could lead to reversible cognitive deficits. Genuine fears such as his ongoing risk of assault were explicitly discussed, and a discharge plan involving moving to a different town broached. Exposure work continued and, as cognition improved, incorporated more cognitive aspects of CBT such as challenging automatic thoughts. Over months his dysphasia resolved, and he was able to function at what his family said was essentially his pre-assault level. Interestingly he still underperformed on formal cognitive testing at this time, especially on executive tasks such as verbal fluency. He described the subjective experience of being overwhelmed and unable to think clearly during cognitive testing.

What Did I Learn from This Case?

This case emphasized the centrality of obtaining accurate information about initial presentation and care, ideally from contemporaneous notes, when assessing any patient with symptoms attributed to brain injury. This is true even in patients who have already received treatment in specialist centers and in whom the diagnosis seems clear. TR's presentation seemed indistinguishable from that of other severely brain-injured patients, and it was only after many weeks of inpatient observations (when there had already been some response to treatment) that inconsistencies in cognitive function were noted by the staff. When it does become clear that cognitive deficits are functional rather than due to brain injury, this must be sensitively but clearly communicated to patients. Delivering therapy and addressing perpetuating factors necessitates multidisciplinary working, in which fairly dramatic social interventions (such as in this case moving to a new town) may be central.

Part IV
Epilepsy and Psychogenic Nonepileptic Seizures

Chapter 20
Novel Seizure Semiology After Epilepsy Surgery

Martin Holtkamp

Summary

A 36-year-old male patient suffers from partial epilepsy since his 8th year of life after – at the age of 5 years – he had fallen out of the window resulting in severe traumatic brain injury. Seizure semiology was stereotypical with tonic posturing of the right upper extremity followed by clonic posturing. Frequency was 4–5 per month. Epilepsy was resistant toward more than 15 common antiepileptic drugs (AED). He received comprehensive work-up for epilepsy surgery and eventually underwent resection of the epileptogenic zone at the posterior margin of the left-hemispheric lesion. Two months postsurgery, he developed fits with a novel semiology. Now, motor signs involved both sides and were fluctuating, eyes were closed, and after movements had ceased, postictally, the patient was immediately reorientated. We diagnosed these paroxysmal events to be psychogenic nonepileptic seizures (PNES) and initiated behavioral psychotherapy. The patient now has been free of epileptic seizures for more than 1 year.

Background Epilepsy History

At age 8 years, the patient started to suffer from monthly epileptic seizures starting with a nonspecific aura and evolution with turning of the head to the right and rhythmic right arm movements without loss of consciousness lasting approximately 2 min. About once a year, these fits develop into generalized tonic-clonic seizures.

M. Holtkamp, MD
Department of Neurology, Epilepsy-Center Berlin-Brandenburg,
Charité – Universitätsmedizin Berlin, Berlin, Germany
e-mail: martin.holtkamp@charite.de

J. Priller, H. Rickards (eds.), *Neuropsychiatry Case Studies*,
DOI 10.1007/978-3-319-42190-2_20

Previously, he failed to respond to anticonvulsant treatment with barbexaclone, carbamazepine, oxcarbazepine, valproic acid, levetiracetam, and lacosamide in adequate doses.

Examination

The patient has some slight mental slowing, but his cognitive functions are otherwise normal. He presents with homonymous hemianopsia to the right and moderate right-sided spastic hemiparesis involving both the upper and lower extremities. Subsequently, his gait is slightly impaired.

Initial and Further Investigations

MRI imaging of the patient's brain showed an extended left-hemispheric lesion with enlarged lateral ventricles and hippocampal volume loss (see Fig. 20.1, left side, upper MRI). Interictal EEG demonstrated a diffuse left-sided slowing with fronto-central-temporal spikes and polyspikes. During video-EEG recordings with scalp electrodes, one seizure was captured. Four seconds before any behavioral changes, an EEG seizure pattern with rhythmic epileptiform discharges was seen left fronto-central-temporally (see Fig. 20.1, right side, upper EEG traces) followed by a forced head and body version to the right and clonic right arm movements which further on evolved to a generalized tonic-clonic seizure. Due to the extent of the lesion and the undefined localization of seizure onset by scalp EEG, subdural strip electrodes were implanted on left frontal, temporal, and parietal brain structures (see Fig. 20.1, left side, lower MRI, position of strip "A" is shown). Two behavioral seizures were recorded, intracranial ictal EEG demonstrated seizure onset with high-amplitude spiking (see Fig. 20.1, right side, lower EEG traces). The white arrow in the lower EEG in Fig. 20.1 indicates seizure onset at electrodes A2 to A4. Latency to first clinical signs was 8 s and thus 4 s longer compared to scalp recordings. Secondary spread of ictal activity to adjacent electrodes occurred within the next 5–10 s.

Therapeutic Procedure and Response to Treatment

Following long-term video-EEG monitoring with intracranial electrodes, tailored cortical resection of brain structures underneath the electrodes A2 to A6 (see Fig. 20.1, left side, lower MRI) and just below the sulcus parallel to the upper posterior margin of the lesion was performed. Six months after the operation, the patient reported two seizures; he was quite frustrated as he felt the resection had

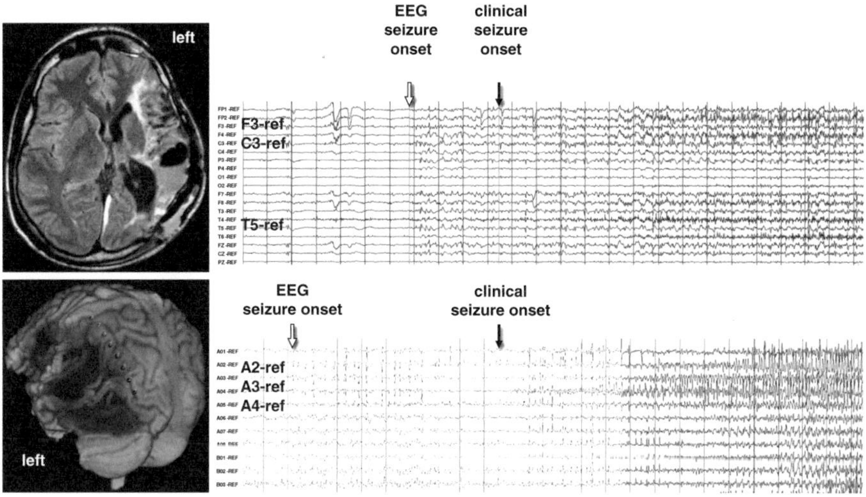

Fig. 20.1 Cranial MRI and EEG traces of a 36-year-old male patient with posttraumatic intractable partial epilepsy. MRI shows a large lesion in the left hemisphere. The lower MRI presents the location of one subdural strip electrode covering the upper and posterior margin of the lesion. The upper EEG traces are recorded by scalp electrodes and the lower by subdural electrodes (Note that the intracranial EEG detects electrophysiological seizure's onset 4 s prior to scalp EEG recordings)

Table 20.1 Characteristics in patients' history and semiological details of psychogenic nonepileptic and epileptic seizures

Features	PNES	Epileptic seizure
Manifestation <10 years of life	Unusual	Common
Recurrent "status"	Common	Rare
Multiple operations/invasive tests	Common	Rare
Psychiatric treatment	Common	Rare
Physical and sexual abuse	Common	Rare
Situational seizure onset	Occasional	Rare
Gradual seizure onset	Common	Rare
Undulating motor activity	Common	Very rare
Rhythmic pelvis movements	Occasional	Rare
"Arc de cercle"	Occasional	Very rare
Closed eyes	Very common	Rare
Convulsions >2 min	Common	Very rare
Rapid postictal reorienting	Common	Unusual

Used with permission from Reuber and Elger [2]

been in vain. On detailed history taking, he said that he had motor signs involving the whole body; this would correspond to tonic-clonic generalized seizures. As increase in seizure severity after epilepsy surgery is rather surprising, we took third-party history by a colleague of the patient. She reported that the patient had been lying on the floor with jerks affecting his upper and lower extremities for 2–3 min.

Motor signs were fluctuating, eyes were closed, and after the end of motor signs, the patient was immediately completely reoriented. During postoperative follow-up of so far 1 year, the patient remained free of any other types of seizures on stable AED medication.

Differential Diagnosis

Failure of epilepsy surgery is seen in approximately 40 % of patients [1]. The more complex the cases, the more likely seizures recur. Therefore, it would not be unlikely that this patient suffers from ongoing seizures after resection of the assumed epileptogenic focus. Description of seizure semiology by the patient was not very helpful to make the correct diagnosis. However, the detailed seizure observation by the patient's colleague clearly indicates PNES. In the current case, typical PNES features include waxing and waning of motor signs, closed eyes, and immediate reorientation. For further features differentiating PNES from epileptic seizures, see Table 20.1 [2]. Incidence of new-onset PNES manifesting after successful epilepsy surgery has recently been described in 4 % of patients [3]. Reported risk factors were female sex and preexisting psychiatric disturbances.

Further Treatment

Just 1 week after we had made the correct diagnosis of PNES, the patient presented to a physician with expertise in psychosomatic medicine specialized on treatment of dissociative disorders. It became obvious that the patient put himself at high pressure regarding his expectations of epilepsy surgery. This may have triggered manifestation of PNES. Since onset of psychotherapy, the patient is free of further psychogenic seizures.

What Did I Learn from This Case?

This neuropsychiatric case presentation offers a couple of interesting learning issues. Firstly, even complex partial epilepsies with lesions due to trauma, infection, neoplasia, or cerebrovascular incidents may successfully undergo epilepsy surgery. Secondly, history taking of third parties is of utmost importance in paroxysmal events such as epileptic seizures as this approach often paves the road to the correct diagnosis. Lastly, not all seizures are of epileptic origin; therefore, always challenge the allegedly nearby diagnosis of epileptic seizures.

References

1. De Tisi J, Bell GS, Peacock JL, McEvoy AW, Harkness WF, Sander JW, Duncan JS. The long-term outcome of adult epilepsy surgery, patterns of seizure remission, and relapse: a cohort study. Lancet. 2011;378:1.388–95.
2. Reuber M, Elger CE. Psychogenic nonepileptic seizures: review and update. Epilepsy Behav. 2013;4:205–16.
3. Markoula S, de Tisi J, Foong J, Duncan JS. De novo psychogenic nonepileptic attacks after adult epilepsy surgery: an underestimated entity. Epilepsia. 2013;54:e159–62.

Chapter 21
The Syndrome of Transient Epileptic Amnesia

Diagnose "Psychogenic" Causation Carefully: Remember That "Standard Tests" Can Sometimes Miss the Point, and Discuss Difficult Cases with Colleagues When in Doubt

Adam Zeman

Case History

A 51-year-old industrial surveyor, KN, presented, many years ago, with a history unlike any I had encountered before. The story was relayed to me by the junior doctor working next door, and, on the first occasion, I met the patient myself only briefly. The history had three main elements. First, for the past year, the patient, KN, had been waking once a month or so in an amnesic state which usually lasted about 20 min. While in this state, he was absolutely unable to remember events from recent days or the tasks of the day ahead. He had partial recollection for the episodes, such that he could, at least to some extent, "remember not being able to remember." Second, independent of the amnesic spells just mentioned, he had noticed that his memory for recent events was fading unusually rapidly over weeks. For example, about 10 weeks before he had spent a fortnight working at a factory which he had not visited before, where he successfully undertook a major survey. By the time of his hospital appointment, although he knew that he had undertaken this piece of work, he had no recollection of the appearance of the factory site or of any of the details of the fortnight he spent there. Thirdly, he had noticed that it had become hard for him to evoke memories of much more distant events, from over 10 years ago, which he knew he could previously recall, including several holidays abroad; he was also finding it hard to recollect previously familiar routes around his familiar neighborhood.

A. Zeman, BA, BM, BCh, DM, FRCP
Cognitive and Behavioural Neurology, University of Exeter Medical School, Exeter, UK
e-mail: a.zeman@exeter.ac.uk

J. Priller, H. Rickards (eds.), *Neuropsychiatry Case Studies*,
DOI 10.1007/978-3-319-42190-2_21

Background History

There were no relevant features in the past medical history. He was taking no medication. KN was a nonsmoker and only moderate drinker. There was, however, a background history of recent stress both at home and work which the general practitioner considered might be relevant to KN's presentation.

Examination

KN was fully cooperative with the assessment and gave an extremely clear account of his symptoms. It seemed unlikely that bedside neurological examination would be helpful, and, indeed, his mini-mental state examination score was 30/30. Neurological examination was also normal.

Initial Diagnosis

The history of recurrent amnesic episodes on awakening, memory "fading" over days to weeks, and apparent loss of previously established memories for events and routes was not familiar to me. Given the "atypical" story, the background of "stress," the normal performance on the MMSE, and the recognized association between memory loss for remote events and "psychogenic" or "functional" amnesia, I initially considered a psychogenic cause a strong possibility in this case. However, in view of the history of episodic symptoms, we organized investigations including an MRI scan of the brain and EEG. I also resolved to discuss the case with my mentor, John Hodges.

Investigation Findings

The MRI scan of the brain was normal, but the EEG revealed frequent spikes originating in the right temporal lobe, suggestive of temporal lobe epilepsy (see Fig. 21.1 for a similar recent example showing recurrent right temporal sharp waves).

Diagnosis

My subsequent conversation with John Hodges about this case introduced me to the recently described syndrome of "transient epileptic amnesia" (TEA). This condition became a research interest for me, and I have since seen well over 100 cases. In this

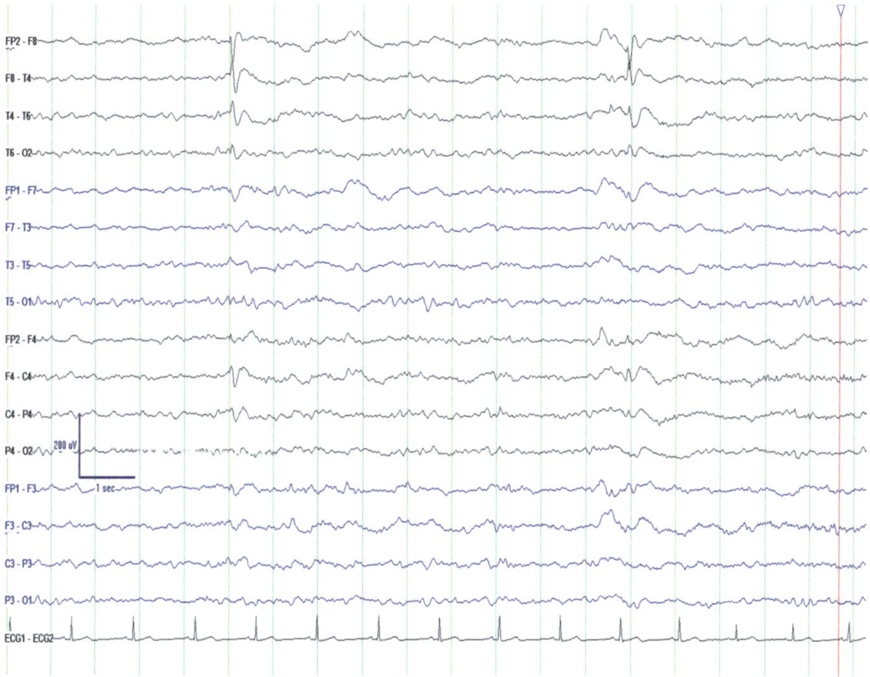

Fig. 21.1 Phase-reversing interictal right temporal lobe sharp waves recorded from a patient with Transient Epileptic Amnesia

condition, the chief and sometimes only manifestation of a temporal lobe seizure is a period of amnesia, typically lasting for less than an hour, often occurring on waking. If there are associated "epileptic" symptoms, these often include olfactory hallucinations. The amnestic episodes of TEA respond well to anticonvulsant drugs as a rule, but there are often persistent, interictal memory problems which respond less well, if at all. These are well illustrated by the case of KN and comprise accelerated long-term forgetting, the loss of memories which appear to have been acquired normally over days to weeks, and remote memory loss, for autobiographical events, routes, and landmarks. Table 21.1 indicates the key features of TEA in contrast to three other causes of transient amnesia, transient global amnesia, transient ischemic amnesia, and psychogenic amnesia.

Follow-Up

After starting on carbamazepine, KN had no further amnestic episodes. His persistent, interictal amnesia was only slightly improved, however, although he remained able to work.

Table 21.1 Differentiating features of transient epileptic amnesia (TEA), transient global amnesia (TGA), transient ischemic amnesia (TIA), and functional amnesia

	TEA	TGA	TIA	Functional
Typical age	50+ years	50+ years	50+ years	Any age
Duration	Typically <1 h	Typically 4–6 h	Variable	Typically days or months
Ictal memory	Variable mix of anterograde and retrograde amnesia – may later remember attack	Dense anterograde amnesia, variable retrograde amnesia	Not well characterized	Variable, but often dense retrograde amnesia (+/– loss of personal identity) with preserved anterograde memory
Other features (sometimes present)	Olfactory hallucinations, automatisms, brief loss of awareness	Headache, nausea	Focal neurological symptoms and signs, usually arising from posterior circulation	Other functional symptoms and signs may be present; mood disturbance
Precipitants	Waking	Physical exertion and/or psychological stress	–	Stressful life events, minor head injury, mood disturbance
Recurrence	Around 1/month	6–10 % recurrence rate/year	Recognized but not well characterized	Unusual but occurs in, e.g., recurrent psychogenic fugue
Past medical history	No established risk factors	Migraine	Cerebrovascular risk factors	Psychiatric illness, "organic" transient amnesia, substance abuse
Interictal/postictal memory	+/– Mild impairment on standard tests; accelerated long-term forgetting, remote memory loss, topographical amnesia	Subtle subclinical impairment may persist for days to months, but no permanent deficit	Risk of permanent memory impairment from completed stroke	Variable

What Did I Learn from This Case?

There are three key learning points. First, I learned to be cautious to attribute symptoms I do not understand to psychogenic or functional disorder. Such "functional" disorders undoubtedly exist and are a central part of neuropsychiatric practice, but they should be diagnosed when there is positive evidence for them, rather than when no better explanation comes to mind. As Thomas Willis wrote in the seventeenth century, such a diagnosis can be the "subterfuge of ignorance." Second, I learned from KN and many subsequent, similar patients that tests should be interpreted thoughtfully. Patients with TEA often perform normally on "standard" tests of memory which examine recall at half an hour. However, this does not imply that their "memory is normal," but rather that the standard tests are failing to measure the problems they are noticing, especially memory loss over longer intervals and autobiographical amnesia. These *can* be measured, but only using appropriate, "nonstandard" tests.

Third, through this case, I discovered a fascinating condition, new to me but not to others, which I continue to research to this day. So the third moral from this case is that it can be enormously helpful to discuss uncertainties with colleagues, especially more experienced and wiser ones. Occasional ignorance is normal, but we owe it to ourselves and to our patients to keep learning whenever we can.

Bibliography

Bartsch T, Deuschl G. Transient global amnesia: functional anatomy and clinical implications. Lancet Neurol. 2010;9:205–14.

Hodges J. Cognitive assessment for clinicians. 2nd ed. Oxford: Oxford University Press; 2007.

Zeman A, Butler C. The syndrome of transient epileptic amnesia. Curr Opin Neurol. 2010;23:610–6.

Zeman A, Kapur N, Jones-Gotman M, editors. Epilepsy and memory. Oxford: Oxford University Press; 2012.

Chapter 22
Autobiographical Amnesia in Association with Subtle Temporal Lobe Seizures

Christopher R. Butler

History

A 31-year-old student of midwifery was referred to the cognitive disorders clinic with a 6-month history of memory problems. She attended the clinic unaccompanied.

She reported being unable to remember important personal events that had occurred over the preceding 5 or 6 years. The problem had first come to light when her husband, a professional photographer, was going through photographs he had taken at the wedding of a family friend about a year previously. She became upset and could not understand why she had not been invited. In fact, however, she *had* been to the wedding and, as proof, her husband showed her photographs in which she appeared. These photographs, however, prompted no recollection of the occasion.

She subsequently realized that there were other salient events of the past few years for which she had no memory. For example, she was unable to recall details about the birth of her third child 3 years previously. She remembered being in hospital and being scheduled for a caesarean section following detection of some reduction in fetal movements, but was unable to remember the birth itself or events of the following few days. Again, photographs taken around the time failed to prompt recollection. As a further example, she described how she had seen a television advertisement for Thailand as a tourist destination and had mentioned to her husband that she would like to visit Thailand one day. Her husband was understandably taken aback, as they had been for a fortnight's holiday 4 years earlier. It emerged that she was unable to remember anything about the trip.

C.R. Butler, MA, MRCP, PhD
Department of Clinical Neurosciences, John Radcliffe Hospital, Oxford, UK
e-mail: chris.butler@ndcn.ox.ac.uk

J. Priller, H. Rickards (eds.), *Neuropsychiatry Case Studies*,
DOI 10.1007/978-3-319-42190-2_22

Despite this problem with remembering past events, the patient claimed to have no difficulty learning new information. She had done exceptionally well in her end of year exams 2 months earlier. She experienced no difficulty remembering recent news events and keeping appointments or with the complex juggling of childcare and her midwifery studies.

The patient had experienced an episode of severe postnatal depression following the birth of her first child, but was successfully treated over a period of 10 months with citalopram and cognitive behavioral therapy. She denied ongoing symptoms of low mood.

Examination

The patient was alert, oriented, and cooperative. She appeared genuinely perplexed by her memory gaps. No abnormality was found on general or neurological examination.

Neuropsychology

Detailed neuropsychometric testing revealed her to have a full-scale IQ of 123. She performed within the "high average" to "superior" range on all tests of anterograde memory, language, attention, executive function, and visuospatial perception. She also performed normally on the autobiographical memory interview, being able to provide a number of detailed memories from her childhood, early adulthood, and recent past. This did not surprise her, since she experienced her autobiographical amnesia as very patchy, with islands of preserved memory in between. The overall clinical impression was that her memory complaints were very unlikely to have a neurological basis and that psychogenic mechanisms, perhaps related to her period of postnatal depression, offered the best explanation of her apparently focal retrograde amnesia.

Follow-Up

One month after her neuropsychological evaluation, she was seen again in clinic, this time in the company of her husband. Interestingly, she claimed to have little or no recollection of the test session, although her husband reported having had a detailed discussion with her about it the day afterward.

Upon direct questioning about ongoing psychiatric symptoms, the patient admitted to experiencing rather frequent panic attacks. These had been occurring once or twice a week over the past 4 years. No consistent triggers were identified and the attacks could even begin when she was sitting quietly watching television. Describing the attacks, she said that she would become overwhelmed with a sensation of déjà vu and a "whooshing feeling," her heart would start racing, and she would feel very hot. If someone spoke to her, it would sound "echoey," but she understood and could respond normally. The sensation typically lasted for a minute or two before spontaneously resolving. The patient's husband confirmed that her appearance during these episodes was normal, although she would sometimes smack her lips as if trying to identify a taste in her mouth.

Further Investigations

The stereotyped attacks of déjà vu and panic raised the suspicion of subtle temporal lobe epilepsy. A routine EEG was unremarkable, but ambulatory monitoring revealed occasional but definite interictal epileptiform discharges over the temporal lobes bilaterally, more pronounced during sleep.

No antibodies associated with autoimmune limbic encephalitis, such as against the voltage-gated potassium channel complex, were detected.

An MRI scan of the head was normal.

Diagnosis

A diagnosis was made of autobiographical amnesia in association with subtle temporal lobe epilepsy.

Management

Antiepileptic therapy with lamotrigine was commenced. This led to an abrupt cessation of the panic/déjà vu episodes. Moreover, the patient later reported that her memory for events that had taken place over the 6 months since starting antiepileptic medication seemed to be better than for events prior to that. No recovery of her memory for more remote autobiographical events was noted.

What Did I Learn from This Case?

This case taught me that loss of remotely acquired autobiographical memories may be the presenting feature of subtle temporal lobe epilepsy.

In organic amnesia, typically arising from damage to the medial temporal lobes, there is usually impairment both of new learning (anterograde amnesia) and of memory for past events (retrograde amnesia). When a patient presents with loss of memories for the past but retains the ability to learn new information, the etiology is often assumed to be "psychogenic." This case indicates that such "focal retrograde amnesia" might instead be caused by subtle epileptic seizures arising from the temporal lobes. As a result, when a patient turns up to clinic complaining of amnesia for past events (typically holidays and weddings), I now always ask about subtle features of epilepsy, such as déjà vu, hallucinations of taste or smell, brief moments of unresponsiveness, or motor automatisms, and have a low threshold for requesting an EEG.

It is interesting to note that the memory complaints of this young patient are very similar to those described by (usually older) people with transient epileptic amnesia (TEA). TEA is a syndrome of epilepsy characterized by recurrent, brief episodes of pure amnesia caused by focal seizures. In between the amnesic attacks, patients with TEA also experience autobiographical amnesia.

Bibliography

Butler CR, Zeman AZ. Recent insights into the impairment of memory in epilepsy: transient epileptic amnesia, accelerated long-term forgetting and remote memory impairment. Brain. 2008;131(Pt 9):2243–63.

Hornberger M, Mohamed A, Miller L, Watson J, Thayer Z, Hodges JR. Focal retrograde amnesia: extending the clinical syndrome of transient epileptic amnesia. J Clin Neurosci. 2010;17(10):1319–21.

Kopelman M. Disorders of memory. Brain. 2002;125(Pt 10):2152–90.

Chapter 23
A Diagnostic Challenge of Troublesome Nocturnal Episodes

Frank Besag

A 7-year-old boy presented with frequent episodes of crying out and screaming at night. His parents commented that the sleep disturbance was affecting the health of the entire family because they could not sleep either.

His early development seemed normal. However, at 5 or 6 months of age, he was less responsive. He stared. He did not appear to be interested in his surroundings. He looked blank much of the time. He put two to three words together with meaning by about 18 months to 2 years of age. His language then regressed between 2 and 3 years of age, when he lost most of the words he had learned. By 2.5 years of age, he had "virtually no language at all." Autism spectrum disorder was diagnosed and it became evident that he had global intellectual disability. The pediatrician was also concerned about "absences." From about 2 years of age, he stared and stopped what he was doing. He did not respond for a few seconds to 2 min. He probably had more than ten episodes daily on most days. An EEG was consistent with a diagnosis of epilepsy. Sodium valproate was commenced. "He started to become more aware of the world." The blank spells were less frequent.

An MRI scan revealed no abnormality.

He attended a special school for children with intellectual disability.

From about 5 years of age, he started having episodes of screaming, shouting, and singing at night. These episodes typically lasted from 1.5 to 2 h but could last for longer. Sometimes they lasted all night.

Carbamazepine was commenced. The nocturnal episodes resolved but he became "sluggish and dopey" during the day. The blank spells were worse. He also fell suddenly, on occasions. Carbamazepine was replaced by sodium valproate. The nocturnal episodes recurred; they became more frequent until they occurred almost every night. Lamotrigine was then commenced. The daytime absence seizures stopped.

F. Besag, BSc, MSc, PhD, MBChB
East London NHS Foundation Trust, Mid Bedfordshire Clinic, Bedford, UK
e-mail: frank.besag@elft.nhs.uk; fbesag@aol.com

J. Priller, H. Rickards (eds.), *Neuropsychiatry Case Studies*,
DOI 10.1007/978-3-319-42190-2_23

His father commented: "It's quite noticeable that since he's been on the lamotrigine, he's been more alert and his language has improved." However, the nocturnal episodes remained troublesome.

When referred to our service at 7 years of age, he was taking sodium valproate 280 mg twice daily and lamotrigine 20 mg twice daily. There were no daytime seizures of any sort. Nocturnal screaming and laughing occurred about six nights a week. He sometimes opened his bowels while he was screaming or laughing at night. The nocturnal shouting/screaming episodes were a major issue and had not responded satisfactorily to the medication he was already taking.

There was no relevant family medical history.

He had an excessive interest in cars and vehicles. He liked routine and wanted things to happen in the right order. He referred to himself by his first name, not using the personal pronouns "I" or "me." His parents did not think that he had any appreciation of other people's feelings or any concept of what other people were thinking. His father commented: "I think he thinks we are thinking what he's thinking."

He presented as a delightful boy who gave good eye contact and established very good rapport. Physical examination revealed no abnormalities.

This case posed the following clinical questions:

1. Why did he lose language between 2 and 3 years of age; does this imply that he has autism?
2. What were the nocturnal episodes?
3. How should he be managed?

These questions will be addressed in turn.

Why did he lose language between 2 and 3 years; does he have autism?

Loss of skills under 3 years of age would be classical for autism. He also exhibited a number of other autistic features, particularly difficulties in interacting with his peers and other people at that time. However, the quality of his social interaction improved markedly following the introduction and adjustment of the antiepileptic drug regime, and epilepsy can also, rarely, be associated with loss of language. Furthermore, subtle manifestations of epilepsy may present as autistic features. His reciprocal social interaction in the clinic setting was good. However, his peer relationships were still not particularly good. The presentation would not be consistent with the classical (Kanner) picture of severe autism, but he had sufficient autistic features for the diagnostic category of "autism spectrum disorder". The apparent improvement in both speech and autistic features with antiepileptic medication might suggest that epilepsy was also playing a role in contributing to the autistic features. The syndrome that is classically associated with speech loss is the Landau-Kleffner syndrome (LKS), but the presentation was not consistent with LKS, which would typically be after speech acquisition (which had barely commenced in this case) and with electrical status epilepticus during slow-wave sleep (ESESS), which none of the EEGs revealed. In this case, the child had global intellectual disability, whereas a child with typical Landau-Kleffner syndrome has specific language impairment. An ambulatory EEG revealed no epileptiform activity; the overnight EEG was performed on one of the few nights when he had no episodes. Previous EEGs had shown a variety of abnormalities but not ESES.

What were the odd nocturnal episodes?

Differential diagnosis of odd nocturnal episodes is very broad. It includes sleepwalking, sleep talking, sleep terrors, sleep starts, hypnagogic and hypnopompic hallucinations, rhythmic movement disorders, restless legs syndrome, periodic limb movements in sleep, confusional arousals, nightmares, and REM sleep behavior disorder.

Nocturnal frontal lobe epilepsy has particularly been brought to the attention of clinicians through the work of Scheffer and colleagues [1] who described the autosomal dominant form of the condition in detail. Although the condition can first present in middle age, the commonest age of presentation is in the first decade of life (53 %) and the second commonest period of presentation is in the second decade of life (35 %). They also described the following features:

Clustering of seizures in 76 %, when several seizures could occur in a single night.
Typically 4–11 attacks (median 6) per night.
Four of their patients commonly had more than 20 seizures per night.
One of their patients had 72 seizures in a single night.
Twenty-four percent reported a single attack per night.

Nearly all the seizures arose from sleep. They commonly occurred soon after falling asleep or as the person dozed, but almost half the patients had attacks in the early hours of the morning, after 4 am. Nine percent reported attacks throughout the night. Thirty percent had seizures during daytime naps. Although 27 % described infrequent attacks while awake, light dozing could not be excluded.

Further features of autosomal dominant nocturnal frontal lobe epilepsy included the following:

Attacks generally brief: estimated duration 5 s to 5 min. Mean timed duration of ictal recordings of five patients was 20 s. An aura occurred in 70 % and woke some individuals.

Clinical characteristics of the seizures described by Scheffer et al. included the following:

Began with a gasp or grunt or vocalization: either a prolonged moan or a single word.
Eyes usually open and staring, sometimes rolled up.

Oral or manual automatisms are uncommon. Motor characteristics of the seizures included thrashing, hyperkinetic activity, tonic stiffening, clonic jerking, sitting up or attempting to sit up, sometimes forced hyperextension which could include grasping the headboard of the bed, head extended and eyes rolled upward, prone, crawling position, felt pushed forward or backward, and some flung out of the bed with injury. It is particularly important to note characteristics that some clinicians might think excluded in the diagnosis of epileptic seizures, including the report that 70 % believed that they were aware during most of the seizures but unable to control their actions and unable to respond, although they could hear and recount events later. Thirty-three percent felt frightened during attacks. Some had fear of falling asleep because of the seizures. Sixty-one percent felt unable to "get one's breath" or that they were choking: objectively these subjects appeared to have difficulty breathing, despite retention of awareness. Thirty-three percent bit their tongue. Thirty percent were incontinent during seizures. Fifty-nine percent had loss of consciousness at some time. Most patients were drowsy after the seizure and fell asleep again. Postictal confusion and headache were rare. The severity of the seizures varied greatly within families. Seizures could occur after a long remission, for example, 10–20 years. The principal trigger factors were stress and fatigue. EEG recordings showed that the attacks were most frequent in stage two sleep but could occur in other stages of non-REM sleep. Six out of 10 of the EEGs showed no ictal changes in the electrographic record.

Many of the characteristics of nocturnal frontal lobe seizures are very different from those usually associated with epileptic seizures. The movements are generally nonrhythmical and may be bizarre, including the flinging about of a single limb or cycling movements of the lower limbs. The fact that patients are generally aware during the seizures, although they have no control over the motor movements, and can remember the episodes afterward might lead many clinicians to exclude epilepsy as a possible diagnosis. As a result, these episodes are often misdiagnosed. Possible misdiagnoses include psychiatric disorders such as hysteria and nocturnal dyskinesias, and, because the subjects often experience a subjective difficulty in breathing, asthma may be incorrectly diagnosed.

Carbamazepine is usually effective for treating nocturnal frontal lobe seizures. The autosomal dominant form of nocturnal frontal lobe epilepsy described by Scheffer and colleagues was the first epilepsy to be linked to a defective gene, coding for the alpha-4 subunit of the neuronal nicotinic acetylcholine receptor, sometimes linked to chromosome 2q13 [2].

How should he be managed?

The episodes had many of the features of nocturnal frontal lobe epilepsy, clustering of attacks, very frequent nocturnal attacks, bizarre nonrhythmical movement, marked vocalization, and response to carbamazepine, although this medication was not tolerated.

Levetiracetam was prescribed. The nocturnal episodes resolved completely and no seizures of any other type were observed. His parents reported that he was sleeping very well: "Quite a dramatic change." His speech improved after the seizure control. He also seemed to be much more attentive. The antiepileptic medication at the time of the seizure control was as follows:

Levetiracetam 125 mg in the morning and 250 mg at night
Lamotrigine 50 mg twice daily
Sodium valproate 280 mg twice daily

Conclusions

The differential diagnosis of odd nocturnal episodes is broad, but nocturnal frontal lobe seizures should be considered if the attacks occur frequently overnight, are associated with vocalization, and involve nonrhythmical, sometimes bizarre, movements. Although investigations can sometimes be very helpful, judgments regarding the treatment of epilepsy are often made largely on clinical grounds, as in this case. Response to antiepileptic medication was very good. In this case, when seizure control was achieved, social interaction and language also improved, emphasizing the importance of appropriate antiepileptic treatment.

References

1. Scheffer IE, Bhatia KP, Lopes-Cendes I, Fish DR, Marsden CD, Andermann E, et al. Autosomal dominant nocturnal frontal lobe epilepsy. A distinctive clinical disorder. Brain. 1995;118(Pt 1):61–73.
2. Phillips HA, Scheffer IE, Berkovic SF, Hollway GE, Sutherland GR, Mulley JC. Localization of a gene for autosomal dominant nocturnal frontal lobe epilepsy to chromosome 20q 13.2. Nat Genet. 1995;10:117–8.

Chapter 24
Past Investigations May Be Misleading

Gregory S. Finucane

GS is a 37-year-old female former clerical worker who had been treated for epilepsy since infancy with no significant periods of remission despite multiple trials of anticonvulsants including phenytoin, carbamazepine, sodium valproate, vigabatrin, gabapentin, lamotrigine, and oxcarbazepine. Her first episode of psychosis was at the age of 26 after commencing topiramate, which was withdrawn. Oxcarbazepine at the age of 27 caused dizzy spells and no useful reduction in seizure frequency and was switched back to carbamazepine. By the age of 28, her seizure frequency was 15 complex partial seizures per month, her mother would not leave her unattended due to wandering, and she was placed on a permanent Invalid's Benefit.

At the age of 29, she became psychotic and aggressive after a seizure that morning, was reassessed by the psychiatrist, found to be delusional, and recommenced on olanzapine. Over the next year, seizures triggered further psychotic episodes and the dose of olanzapine was increased. She also trialed quetiapine, risperidone, and ziprasidone. Trials of lamotrigine (again), oxcarbazepine, and lacosamide were not successful, and levetiracetam was beneficial for a year and then seizures recurred and depression became more of an issue. There was a complex interaction between seizures, delusional material, anxiety, and low mood, and it was becoming less clear which episodes were epileptic and which were not. In particular frequent "background seizures" were being considered possible anxiety attacks or withdrawal phenomena related to her benzodiazepine use.

G.S. Finucane, MBChB, MA, FRANZCP
Auckland City Hospital, Auckland, New Zealand
e-mail: GFinucane@adhb.govt.nz

J. Priller, H. Rickards (eds.), *Neuropsychiatry Case Studies*,
DOI 10.1007/978-3-319-42190-2_24

Background History

She left school at the age of 18, not achieving a higher qualification, and then became a receptionist and worked in various clerical roles until age 26. After the first psychotic episode, her return to work was not successful and she has continued living with her parents.

Previous Investigations

When investigated at age 17 with bilateral foramen ovale electrodes and video-EEG monitoring, she was found to have seizures arising from both temporal lobes independently, and MR scanning showed increased T2 signal in the right anterior hippocampus. When surgery was reconsidered at age 28, there was a very active focus in the left temporal lobe, probable right hippocampal atrophy, and increased signal but no other change posteriorly in the left hippocampus (Fig. 24.1a, b). We decided that surgery was not indicated as she would be at risk for significant memory impairment, along with persisting seizures from the contralateral temporal lobe.

Progress

She presented acutely after deliberate self-harm with an 8 in. knife, in a psychotic state precipitated by a cluster of partial seizures. Believing that she was Mary and now pregnant with the Devil's child, she had made 13 stab wounds to her anterior abdomen (breaching peritoneum) and anterior chest. Bilateral pneumothoraces and small bowel injury were repaired, and her antipsychotic medication adjusted.

The epilepsy service was greatly perturbed by this event and combination of refractory seizures and relapsing psychosis; as it was recognized, this could easily prove fatal in the next few years. As she had used all available anticonvulsant medication with no benefit, surgical treatment for her epilepsy was reconsidered as it might prove possible to resect the right temporal lobe if the problematic simple partial seizures continued to arise from there. Removing her speech-dominant left temporal lobe, however, would not be considered. Thus, she underwent repeat MRI imaging and repeat video monitoring.

Reinvestigation

The video-EEG monitoring showed bilateral independent epileptiform discharges during sleep, and a "background seizure" during the day was not associated with EEG changes. However the only actual clinical and electroencephalographic complex partial seizure arose from the left temporal region. Attempted ictal SPECT was not successful. While the MRI scan performed at age 28 had been reported to show bilateral hippocampal sclerosis, the repeat imaging one decade later showed a shrunken left posterior hippocampus together with no new changes in the right hippocampus (Fig. 24.2a, b).

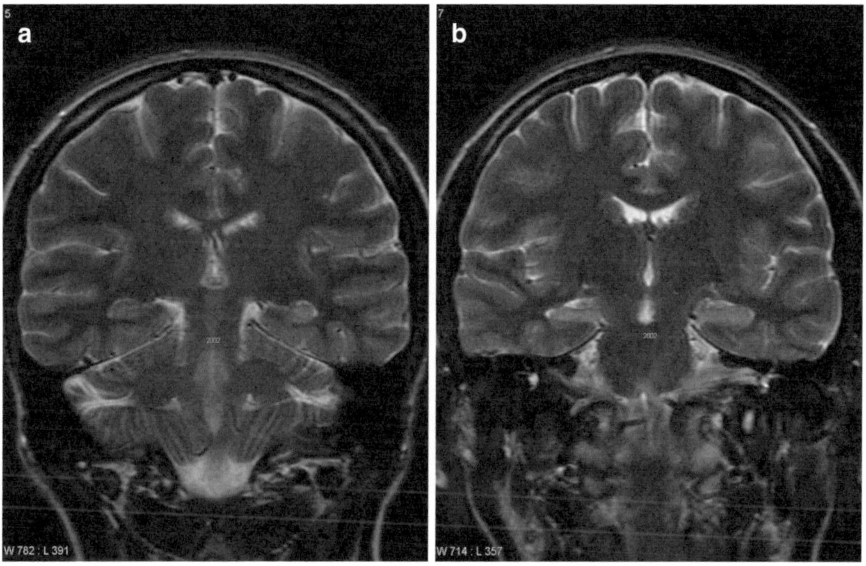

Fig. 24.1 (**a**, **b**) MR slices through hippocampi, one decade apart

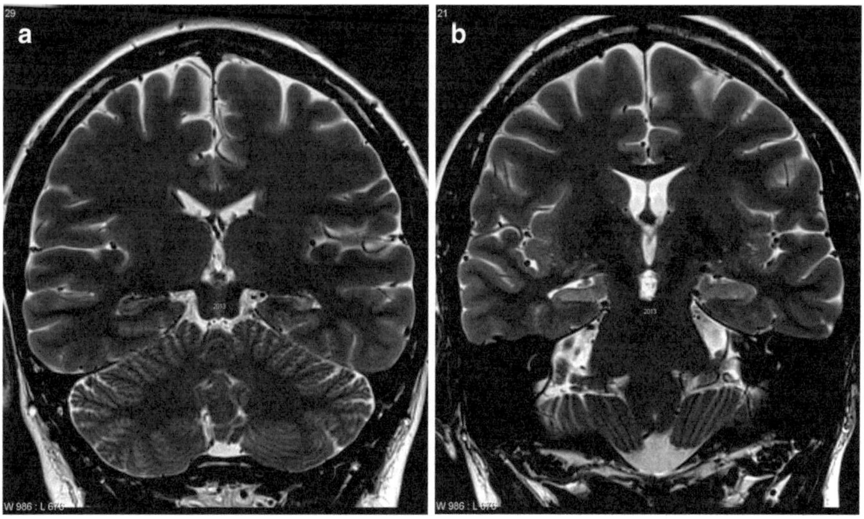

Fig. 24.2 (**a**, **b**) MR slices through hippocampi, one decade apart

Management and Outcome

Once all evidence was reviewed, the epilepsy service concluded that the problematic seizures were largely left sided and that, as the left hippocampus had become much more abnormal over time, a left temporal lobectomy would be feasible after all. There was considerable trepidation given that we had not previously proposed temporal lobectomy for an individual with frequent psychotic phenomena.

She proceeded to stealth-guided left temporal lobectomy with partial amygdalo-hippocampectomy and, by 2 weeks later, had not had any major complex partial seizures. The postoperative stay was uncomplicated, with no seizure activity whilst in the hospital, though she developed a mild expressive and receptive dysphasia. She had an occasional unusual thought that passed through her head, which might be a brief aura but would disappear immediately. Her wound healed well.

At 6 months, the history was of only a handful of complex partial seizures since the operation, and despite unusual cognitions at times for which she took just 25 mg quetiapine prn and simple partial seizures with forced thinking, there has been no further self-harm, no persisting depression (on venlafaxine 37.5 mg daily), and episodes of anxiety only when fatigued. Any brief psychotic experiences had been short lived and easily managed, the dysphasia largely resolved, and she was forming friendships and engaging in voluntary work.

What Did I Learn from This Case?

There were several important lessons from this case. One was that medial temporal sclerosis is a progressive disease [1] and that one cannot therefore rely on the results of remote investigations, which may eventually become misleading. Another is that neither psychosis nor bilateral disease is an absolute contraindication to temporal lobectomy. Surgery can be an effective treatment for psychosis in this setting, despite the evidence base being insecure [2], and there apparently being no internationally agreed standard for neuropsychiatric contraindications to temporal lobectomy.

Bibliography

1. Berg AT. The natural history of mesial temporal lobe epilepsy. Curr Opin Neurol. 2008;21:173–8.
2. Farooq S, Sherin A. Interventions for psychotic symptoms concomitant with epilepsy. Cochrane Database Syst Rev. 2012;2008(4):Art No CD 006118.
3. Marchetti RL, et al. Complete remission of epileptic psychosis after temporal lobectomy. Arq Neuro-Psiquiatr. 2001;59(no.3B).

Chapter 25
New Type of Paroxysmal Events in a Patient with Epilepsy and Learning Difficulties

Maria (Meritxell) Oto

BM is a 20-year-old lady with moderate learning difficulties, autism, challenging behavior, and a diagnosis of epilepsy since the age of 3.

Over the previous 8 months, the family had been aware of a new type of paroxysmal event. They first observed these new events after BM returned home following a period of respite, and initially they thought she was copying behaviors that she had observed at her respite unit (this had occurred on previous occasions).

Events occurred exclusively at mealtimes. Although BM had always focused on mealtimes and a degree of agitation was sometimes associated with this, the new events occurred on a daily basis and at a level of disturbance that was unprecedented. There was no response to behavioral or psychotropic drug intervention, and BM was referred to the Scottish Epilepsy Centre for further assessment.

Description of New Type of Events

The events were generally at the evening or less often at the midday meal. The onset was always shortly after she began to eat. Initially she may pick up a fork and try and insert it in her mouth or start muttering "mum," looking vacant with a fixed smile. She would then repeatedly put her finger in her mouth to the point of gagging and retching. If she were not removed from the dining table, her behavior would escalate to extreme distress, shouting, and hitting out for up to 30 min. However, if taken to her room to lie down, she might continue to put her finger into her mouth for a few minutes, but the event then subsides and she is able to return to finish her meal.

M. Oto, LGMS, PhD, MECPsych
Department of Neuropsychiatry, Scottish Epilepsy Centre, Glasgow, UK
e-mail: meritxelloto@hotmail.com

J. Priller, H. Rickards (eds.), *Neuropsychiatry Case Studies*,
DOI 10.1007/978-3-319-42190-2_25

Background History

BM was born through normal delivery; as a baby she had some feeding difficulties and choking episodes. By the age of 3, she was found to have global developmental delay. Some features were consistent with Prader-Willi syndrome but genetic test did not confirm this.

In terms of her epilepsy, she started having obvious seizures at 3 years of age. The seizures would start with some movement of her trunk, she would then look blank, and eyes deviate to the left for a few seconds. She continues to have this type of seizure occasionally.

Nocturnal seizures began at age 7. She would suddenly sit up in bed with extension and posturing of both arms and some rocking of the upper body and would appear to retch toward the end. These events would last less than a minute. BM has not had any of these events since the introduction of lamotrigine 3 years ago.

BM had a 24 h EEG 2 years ago, which showed pronounced generalized slow-wave abnormalities, which were often rhythmical and sometimes sharp. No obvious seizures were recorded.

Differential Diagnosis

One possibility was that these were behavioral events. In favor would be the fact that BM has had challenging behavior throughout her life, sometimes centered on food. In addition, the events seemed too long for an epileptic seizure, at time lasting over 30 min, and did not seem to respond to a trial of topiramate or diazepam 5 mg twice daily.

However, "eating epilepsy" is a rare type of reflex epilepsy where seizures are triggered by the act of eating [2, 3]. BM is known to have epilepsy, these new events were reasonably stereotyped, and one of the features, retching, had been also present as part of BM's nocturnal events.

Further Investigation

BM was admitted for a period of assessment to the Scottish Epilepsy Centre. Specifically this made available the option of ambulatory video EEG, the only type of investigation that BM could tolerate for any length of time.

Within 24 h two events were captured during eating which were recognized by her carers as typical. These were unequivocally epileptic with a change in behavior associated with a prolonged period of significant EEG slowing and repetitive high-amplitude complexes of variable frequency seen bilaterally. Electrical onsets and offsets are insidious and support a prolonged ictal phase – 16 min in 1 and 22 min in the other. Subclinical seizure activity is noted at other times, but no clear clinical seizures were captured when she was not sitting eating a meal. See Figs. 25.1a, b, 25.2a, b, and 25.3a, b.

Diagnosis

The diagnosis of eating epilepsy was made based on the history, semiology of events, and, crucially in this case, abnormal EEG during the episodes.

Lacosamide was added to her other anticonvulsants and led to the subsequent reduction in frequency and intensity of events.

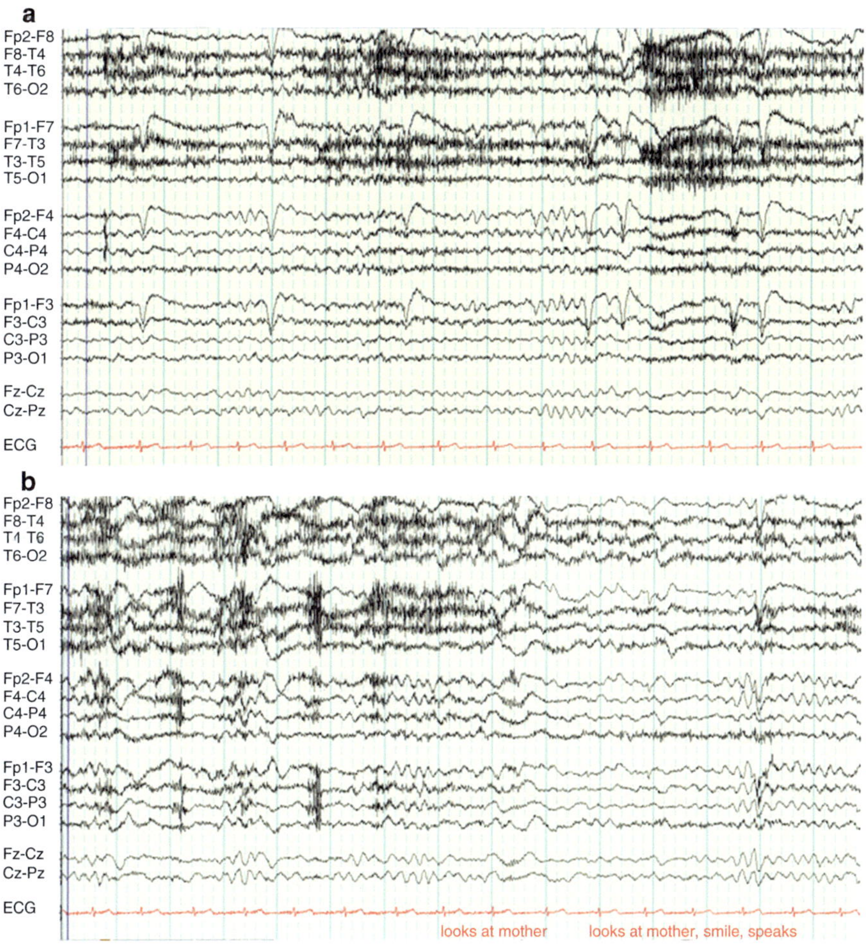

Fig. 25.1 (**a**, **b**) Before the event

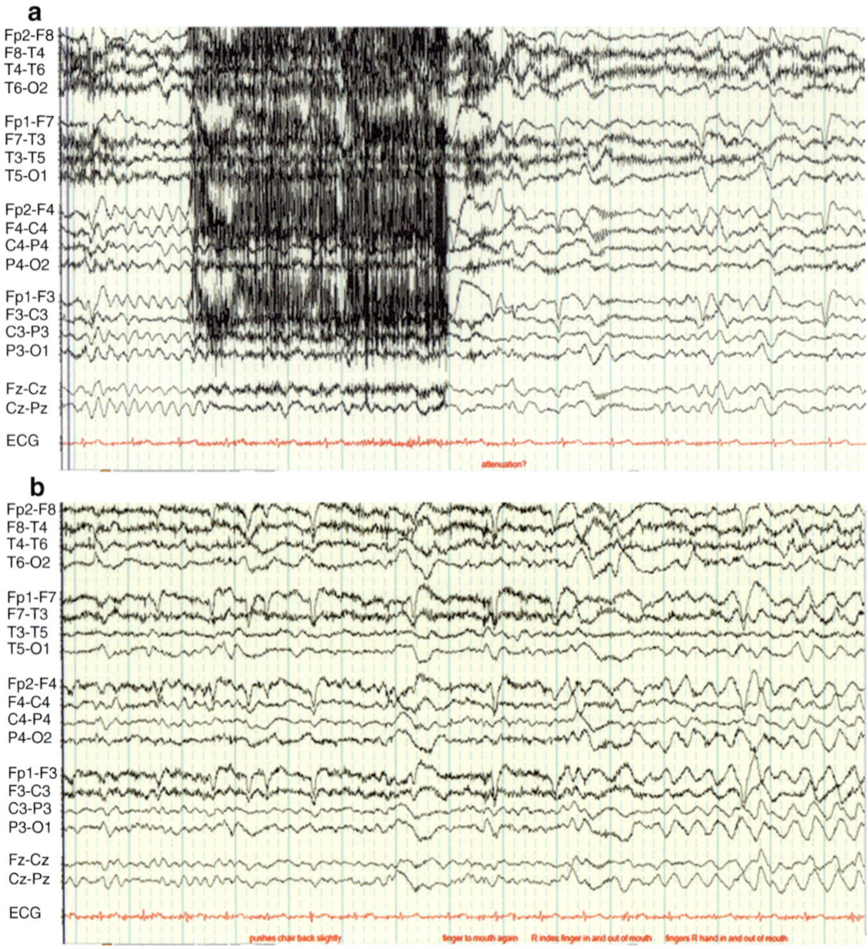

Fig. 25.2 (**a**, **b**) Clinical onset

The family felt greatly relieved to have an explanation for events that had caused extraordinary disruption and distress over preceding months.

What Did I Learn from This Case?

Patients with learning disabilities, epilepsy, and behavioral problems pose diagnostic challenges that can lead to both under- and overdiagnosis [1]. In this case, persistence with failed trials of behavioral, psychotropic, and empirical anticonvulsant medication without a clear diagnosis led to an unwarranted delay in effective treatment. Although the diagnosis of eating epilepsy is rare, ambulatory video EEG is a noninvasive and

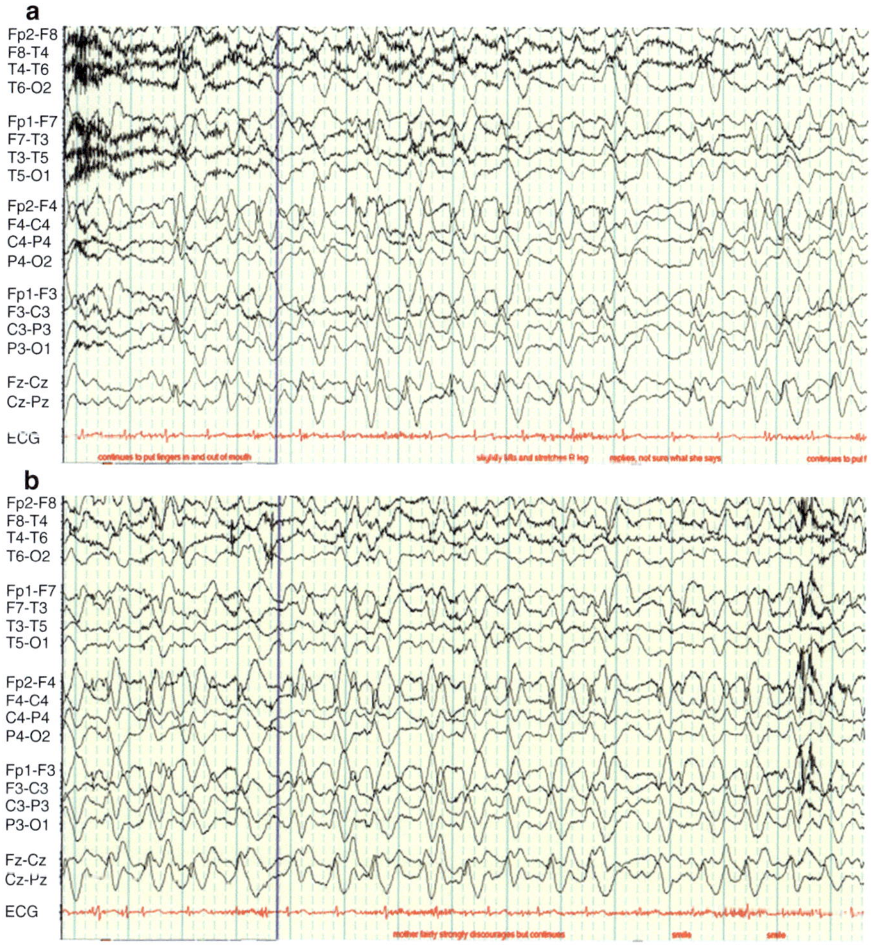

Fig. 25.3 (**a**, **b**) During the event

relatively easily performed test and should have been employed in preference to a series of time-consuming and fruitless therapeutic trials in various modalities.

References

1. Chapman M, Iddon P, Atkinson K, Brodie C, Mitchell D. The misdiagnosis of epilepsy in people with intellectual disabilities: a systematic review. Seizure. 2011;20(2):101–6.
2. Patel M, Satishchandra P, Saini J, Bharath RD, Sinha S. Eating epilepsy: phenotype, MRI, SPECT and video-EEG observations. Epilepsy Res. 2013;107:115–20.
3. Kokes U, Baykan B, Babek N, Gurses C. Eating epilepsy is associated with initial precipitating events and therapy resistance. Clin EEG Neurosci. 2013;44(2):161–6.

Chapter 26
Is Less Really More? The Pitfalls of an Ambitiously Healthy Diet

Marion Lautenschlager

A 48-year-old computer administrator, who lived alone with no history of alcohol abuse, grew confused over a couple of days until his mother found him in his flat, where he was recovering from the first epileptic seizure of his life, still quite disoriented and mutistic. On the way to the hospital, he suffered another grand mal seizure in the ambulance, which was well documented by the accompanying physician.

Background

After an unremarkable early life with successful university studies in computer science and later working in the profession as an IT administrator, he developed his first episode of paranoid schizophrenia at the age of 26, with symptoms of anxiety, feeling observed, hearing voices, and further on with a tendency of avoiding contact to people and staying indoors. There was no history of alcohol or drug abuse and he did not develop any either. He was admitted to a psychiatric hospital almost once a year during the next 9 years and treated with flupentixol long-lasting injections, later with oral risperidone. At the age of 37, he received a disability pension. Under risperidone long-lasting injections, he finally grew stable without any residual positive symptoms of schizophrenia. Only negative symptoms remained (deficits in concentration, cognitive tempo, and flexibility), and he successfully developed a routine of meeting with friends to play bridge and visiting a community center twice a week. He stayed single but frequently visited his nearby living mother and had a fondness for her cooking.

M. Lautenschlager, MD, Dipl Chem
Department of Neuropsychiatry, Charité – Universitätsmedizin Berlin, Berlin, Germany
e-mail: marion.lautenschlager@charite.de

J. Priller, H. Rickards (eds.), *Neuropsychiatry Case Studies*,
DOI 10.1007/978-3-319-42190-2_26

Under the medication with risperidone, and later with added mirtazapine to reduce symptoms of sleeplessness, he gradually developed obesity and type II diabetes, which he found shameful. Medication was switched to ziprasidone, and he remained stable with regard to schizophrenia. He tried to reduce his weight and succeeded to at least stop further weight gain. Then he was persuaded by financial benefits to participate in a health insurance program, which coaches patients with early type II diabetes to achieve goals in weight reduction and a healthy lifestyle. He started going for extensive walks and skipping meals, and he soon discovered (and was coached to do so by the program) that eating less can best be achieved by drinking lots of sugar-free fluids like teas, mineral water, or sugar-free soft drinks. He was proud to lose 10 kg of weight within a couple of months, and his diabetes was so well under control by then that he did not require any oral antihyperglycemic medication anymore. He still appreciated his mother's home cooking at least twice a week when he visited her, but fixed only small meals for himself at home, consisting of pasta dishes or bread with ham and raw vegetables like salted tomatoes.

A year after starting the program, he was still stable with regard to schizophrenia (no positive symptoms), but he developed a chronic bowel disorder with daily bouts of intense flatulence and a piercing pain in his abdomen. The latter grew so intense that he went to the hospital, where he was admitted to a surgical ward. The ultrasound and CT diagnostics showed inflammation of the lower bowels, which was considered to be a case of epiploic appendagitis, an inflammation caused either by torsion of an epiploic appendage or spontaneous venous thrombosis of a draining appendageal vein. Approximately 7 % of patients investigated to exclude sigmoid diverticulitis have imaging findings of primary epiploic appendagitis [1]. He was put on parenteral nutrition with analgesics, antibiotics, and anti-inflammatory drugs for 2 weeks and got better. In the following years, he was twice readmitted to the surgical ward of the hospital with the same symptoms, and diverticulitis of the sigma was diagnosed, and an epiploic appendix of the sigma was extirpated. Preoperatively, the fierce bowel pain had already decreased under treatment with laxatives. During the next one and a half years, no spectacular pain occurred anymore, but he regularly experienced flatulence and milder pain of the bowels. He gradually developed gout (which was treated with allopurinol) and benign hyperplasia of the prostate (which was treated with tamsulosin), as well as arterial hypertonia (which was treated with diuretics).

He tolerated these hospital treatments for bowel disease without further exacerbations of his schizophrenia. He then suffered a major setback at age 47 when his mother had a serious car accident and was diagnosed with cancer a short while later, but she recovered over a time span of several months. He did not suffer from an exacerbation of schizophrenia but did avoid unnecessary outings from his flat or trips to unaccustomed places, as he was wary of the risks of traffic. In this time, he received help from an assertive community treatment team (ACT team) from the local mental health service. The community nurse, among other activities, regularly cooked vegetable stews with him at home twice a week, as his mother was still reconvalescent. On such days, his bowel symptoms were much better. He appreciated the company a lot and thought his reduced bowel problems must result from having meals together. His mother eventually recovered and the visits of the ACT team stopped. The frequency of contact could be reduced again to the appointments with his psychiatrist once a month, as before. Then, without any obvious cause, he grew confused over a couple of days and suffered an epileptic seizure for the first time in his life.

Examination

Upon admission to the hospital after suffering two epileptic seizures, he was disoriented and answered only scarcely to questions with a slurred speech. He seemed distrustful of any intended interventions by the treating physicians. He showed no cranial nerve symptoms and no pathological reflexes. No weakness or changes in muscle tone were present. His gait was ataxic and coordination aberrant, without side differences. He showed no signs of sensory deficit.

Initial Investigations

Cranial MRI was normal but the laboratory results showed marked hyponatremia. Other investigations along the differential diagnosis of epilepsy and his other preexisting conditions were normal (parameters of the liver, kidney, pancreas, thyroid, heart, vitamins, glucose, uric acid, proteins, blood panel, CRP, temperature). No intoxication of any sort was detected. Tests for porphyria were done 2 days after the seizures and turned out normal. He improved after 3 days in the hospital and was released with the recommendation of elective endocrinological evaluation.

Progress

In the meantime, he saw his psychiatrist and admitted to chronic abuse of laxatives once every 3 weeks since he had found out that his bowel pain could be reduced by laxatives. In addition, he reported that his bowel symptoms tended to occur less when he ate less, so he had developed the habit of eating mainly fruit or salted tomatoes, sometimes yoghurt, and drinking up to 6 l of water per day. The harmful consequences of such a chronic unbalanced diet and polydipsia were discussed with him and with his mother, and he promised to return to a normal diet.

He was admitted to the endocrinology ward, and the laboratory testing revealed normal results for testosterone, human-luteinizing hormone, follicle-stimulating hormone, prolactin, insulin-like growth hormone, IGF1-SDS, ACTH, SHBG (IESL), cortisol at different times of the day, ACTH-NN, TSH, fT3, fT4, as well as several electrolytes' (Na, K, Ca, Phos, Cl) osmolality, extended renal parameters, and extended protein and blood panel. An ultrasound of the suprarenal gland was normal. Also the hyponatremia had returned to low normal (137 mmol/l) levels. Finally, the diagnosis of SIADH (syndrome of inappropriate antidiuretic hormone secretion) was suggested, possibly under antipsychotic medication with ziprasidone for psychosis and medication with chloral hydrate for insomnia. His admitted polydipsia was taken into consideration for the hyponatremia, and the abuse of laxatives was considered causal for his bowel symptoms due to painful obstipation.

In spite of his best intentions, the patient returned to the previous habit of polydipsia and fasting after the bowel symptoms reoccurred. He was admitted to a psychiatric ward to restore a normal diet. Although he showed no clear symptoms of exacerbation of schizophrenia, he grew mistrustful of questions about his eating habits, and he wished to leave after a few days of lab tests (all normal). He mentioned an appointment for cataract surgery as the reason for leaving the hospital. He was released with the conviction of the staff that his polydipsia might be related to paranoid symptoms and/or sensations of coenaesthesia due to schizophrenia. Especially his very imperious claim that the sensation of "a ring of fire in his upper bowels" was not being dealt with to his expectations was interpreted as hypochondriac delusion.

Differential Diagnosis

At this point, it was clear that the patient suffered from recurring marked hyponatremia. He admitted to drinking up to 6 l of tap water per day, when his perceived bowel symptoms were more than he could tolerate. This led to the possible diagnosis of PIP syndrome (psychosis, hyponatremia, and polydipsia), which is not uncommon. Seventy percent of chronic psychiatric patients show symptoms of disturbed homeostasis, and 6.6 % of hospitalized patients in a study by Jose et al. [2] had a history of compulsive water intake. Most of the 15.7 % of mentally ill patients, who showed primary polydipsia in a prospective study of an outpatient population, were not aware of the severity and possible complications of such behavior [3]. Lydakis et al. [4] reported a case that presented with epileptic seizures as the first symptom of polydipsia.

A second possible diagnosis was medication-induced SIADH syndrome. A considerable number of substances have been associated with this disorder, among them (*underlined* the ones he had taken over the years): antidepressants (tricyclic and SSRIs, including *mirtazapine*), antipsychotics (mainly phenothiazines like thioridazine, and butyrophenones like *haloperidol*, but also *risperidone*), antiepileptics like carbamazepine and valproate, *antidiabetic drugs*, antihypertonic drugs like *nifedipine* or *amlodipine* or ACE inhibitors, nonsteroidal anti-inflammatory drugs like *ibuprofen* or *paracetamol*, as well as several *antibiotics* [5, 6]. Porphyria, tumors of the suprarenal cortex, and intracranial processes were excluded.

Further Progress and Investigations

Although his schizophrenia was stable, several different medication regimes (including aripiprazole, amisulpride, and combinations with ziprasidone, including added pregabalin) were tried in our patient in order to reduce the possible causes of hyponatremia. His schizophrenia remained stable, but no changes in his perceived bowel symptoms and the habit of polydipsia were achieved outside a hospital ward. Eventually, he refused to set foot in a psychiatric ward again, because he felt that he was not taken seriously by the staff during his most recent stay.

After a series of epileptic seizures, he was admitted the next year to the hospital with bilateral humerus fractures. Porphyria tests were done in the acute state and turned out normal. After recovery and rehabilitation, he suffered a status epilepticus about a year later. He was found at home unconscious with an aspiration pneumonia after having vomited and with multiple fractures of the left ileum and acetabulum. During the lengthy hospital stay, his psychiatrist visited him on the ward. After inquiring about his bowel symptoms, he responded that he suffered from the flatulence and pain in the hospital only after breakfast and supper, but never after lunch.

Diagnosis

After discussing the content of his meals, the best guess seemed to be an intolerance for the bread in every hospital breakfast and supper. He was fine with milk products at home and during hospital lunch so that lactose intolerance could be excluded. He did not test positive for celiac disease serology but seemed to show the symptoms of wheat intolerance. So NCGS (non-celiac gluten sensitivity, synonymous with non-celiac wheat sensitivity) was the hypothesis upon which he began a low-wheat diet. This disease, which is only diagnosed by exclusion of celiac disease and other bowel disorders, has been associated with wheat amylase trypsin inhibitors [7] and shown to improve under reduction of wheat/gluten intake [8]. Our patient's bowel disorder improved significantly mainly by avoiding pasta dishes and wheat in his bread, and with the reduced pain, he was able to stop his habit of fasting and his almost fatal habit of polydipsia. Hyponatremia did not occur anymore. And finally, he was very happy to have a diagnosis other than PIP syndrome to explain his ordeals, in spite of having to live with an only partially recovered mobility after the series of fractures.

What Did I Learn from This Case?

It was interesting to observe that all community-based mental health professionals who knew him well over several years (psychiatrist, nurses, sociotherapist) were looking for a rare neurological or systemic disease to explain his problems. They could not accept PIP-syndrome with its suggestion of a delusion-based causality as the explanation, because they knew his schizophrenia to have been stable for years. In contrast the hospital intern professionals who did not know him well (psychiatrist, nurses, therapists) were satisfied with this diagnosis and even started to interpret his real sensations as delusional as well, which drove him further from trusting them. I learned from this patient that voluntary polydipsia in combination with fasting can result in potentially life-threatening seizures and fractures. Especially the chronic mild hyponatremia is associated with a secondary osteoporosis and a higher liability to bone fractures during an epileptic seizure [9]. And the mental symptoms of chronic hyponatremia (mood swings, attention deficits, unsteadiness, and falls) can easily be confused with symptoms of schizophrenia and thus be misinterpreted [10]. Finally, I learned to respect the potential health risks of nutrition intolerances in our patients. When we step into a supermarket today and contemplate the endless rows of lactose-free, gluten-free, and wheat-free products, or other food deprived of specified ingredients, we like to consider this to be merely a smart marketing fashion, and we tend to ask ourselves whether any of these supposed intolerances would be detectable by scientific means. But this patient taught me that it is irrelevant whether he succeeds in convincing us doctors that his perceived bowel disturbances are severe enough to justify an additional IDC10 diagnosis. What is highly relevant, however, is whether he considers the bowel troubles intolerable enough to justify extreme actions on his part to avoid their occurrence. So we are well advised to take our time to discuss possible healthy diet options for perceived symptoms of our patients in order to prevent escalations of the described type. And once in a while, it is really just plain pasta or naturally baked bread causing the havoc, and not the prescribed, pharmaceutically manufactured medication, which is so frequently being considered the culprit.

Bibliography

1. Subramaniam R. Acute appendagitis: emergency presentation and computed tomographic appearances. Emerg Med J. 2006;23:e53.
2. Jose CJ, Perez-Cruet J. Incidence and morbidity of self-induced water intoxication in state mental hospital patients. Am J Psychiatry. 1979;136:221–2.
3. Iftene F, Bowie C, Milev R, Hawken E, Talikowska-Szymczak E, Potopsingh D, Hanna S, Mulroy J. Identification of primary polydipsia in a severe and persistent mental illness outpatient population: a prospective observational study. Psychiatry Res. 2013;210:679–83.
4. Lydakis C, Apostolakis S, Thalassinos E, Stamataki K, Saridaki K, Basta M. PIP syndrome: a potentially threatening manifestation of a psychiatric disorder. J Clin Pract. 2005;59(5):612–3.
5. Liamis G, Milionis H, Elisaf M. A review of drug-induced hyponatremia. Am J Kidney Dis. 2008;52:144–53.
6. Verbalis JG, Goldsmith SR, Greenberg A, Korzelius C, Schrier RW, Sterns RH, Thompson CJ. Diagnosis, evaluation, and treatment of hyponatremia: expert panel recommendations. Am J Med. 2013;126:S1–42.

7. Junker Y, Zeissig S, Kim SJ, Barisani D, Wiesner H, Leffler DA, Zevallos V, Libermann TA, Dillon S, Freitag TL, Kelly CP, Schuppan D. Wheat amylase trypsin inhibitors drive intestinal inflammation via activation of toll-like receptor 4. J Exp Med. 2012;209:2395–408.
8. Carrocio A, Mansueto P, Iacono G, Soresi M, D'Alcamo A, Cavataio F, Brusca I, Florena AM, Ambrosiano G, Sedita A, Pirrone G, Rini GB. Non-celiac wheat sensitivity diagnosed by double-blind placebo-controlled challenge: exploring a new clinical entity. Am J Gastroenterol. 2012;107:1898–906.
9. Kinsella S, Moran S, Sullivan MO, Molloy MCM, Eustace JA. Hyponatremia independent of osteoporosis is associated with fracture occurrence. Clin J Am Soc Nephrol. 2010;5(2):275–80.
10. Renneboog B, Wusch W, Vandemergel X, Manto MU, Decaux G. Mild chronic hyponatremia is associated with falls, unsteadiness, and attention deficits. Am J Med. 2006;119:71.e1–8.

Part V
Metabolic Disorders and Autoimmune Encephalopathies

Chapter 27
Neurometabolic Conditions May Coexist with Symptoms of Autism

Susan Byrne and Tammy Hedderly

Background History

The patient was born at term to consanguineous parents. He showed signs of global developmental delay in the first few years of life. He did not sit alone until 15 months and walked aged 2 years. He did not have single words until 4 years. Communication skills were limited, and he was described as a quiet boy who preferred his own company. The boy developed obsessional play, repetitive behavior, and echolalia and was formally diagnosed by the community pediatric team with autism spectrum disorder (ASD) aged 5 years. The assessments done included interviews and using standardized tools with an Autism Diagnostic Observation Schedule (ADOS).

At 10 years of age, he was referred to the community child and adolescent mental health team, as he developed oppositional behavior that was difficult to manage, and he was noted to have become more quiet and withdrawn. Issues with sudden-onset fecal soiling subsequently emerged. There was a short hospital admission for diarrhea in the same period, and intravenous rehydration was required. Viral gastroenteritis was diagnosed. Mildly abnormal liver function tests were documented during this admission but not investigated. At the age of 11 years, he had a single episode of focal posturing considered to have been a possible seizure. MRI and EEG carried out after this episode were reported to be normal.

A 10-year-old boy with a diagnosis of autism spectrum disorder was referred to the community child and adolescent mental health team, with worsening oppositional behavior, which was difficult to manage.

S. Byrne, MB, BAO, BCh, PhD, MRCPI, MRCPCH
Paediatric Neurology, Evelina Children's Hospital, St. Thomas' Hospital, London, UK
e-mail: susan.byrne@gstt.nhs.uk

T. Hedderly, MBBS, BSc (Hons), FRPCH (✉)
Evelina London Children's Hospital and St Thomas' Hospital, London, UK
e-mail: tammy.hedderly@gstt.nhs.uk

J. Priller, H. Rickards (eds.), *Neuropsychiatry Case Studies*,
DOI 10.1007/978-3-319-42190-2_27

Around this age, his parents had noted a left-sided tremor following antibiotic therapy with penicillin for tonsillitis.

The boy then significantly regressed over the next year in his language skills, and he was reported to be clumsy and less steady on his feet. His parents also noted unusual episodes of freezing lasting for up to an hour. He had an increasing frequency of nosebleeds. During this time, his behavior was becoming increasingly oppositional.

He was then referred to the neurology department aged 12 years having presented acutely with "being off his legs" with a history of deteriorating gait. Since admission, he had reduction in speech output and abnormal movement with catatonic posturing.

Examination (While in the Hospital)

The boy was not dysmorphic. He was mildly icteric and some bruising was noted on his skin. Up-gaze was markedly reduced; however, fundoscopy was normal. He was not very interactive, but his parents commented this was not unusual for him. He had a mild action tremor bilaterally and some parkinsonian features of bradykinesia and rigidity. He was nonverbal and had poor eye contact. Reflexes were brisk throughout. The liver was palpable at 1 cm below the costal margin.

Initial Investigation

MRI brain (Fig. 27.1) was repeated and was supportive of the diagnosis of Wilson's disease. Liver function tests were abnormal and suggestive of chronic liver disease, vitamin K was low, and clotting factors were deranged. There was pancytopenia with evidence of splenomegaly on abdominal ultrasound. Ophthalmology examination confirmed Kayser-Fleischer rings which are seen in Wilson's disease (Fig. 27.2a, b).

Diagnosis

The diagnosis of Wilson's disease was confirmed as ceruloplasmin was low. The liver biopsy confirmed the diagnosis with focal deposits of copper-binding protein and high copper levels. Mutation analysis confirmed a genetic mutation.

Progress

The boy was commenced on penicillamine; however, the response was minimal and the tremor and catatonic symptoms worsened. Therapy was changed to trientine, and an improvement in neurological examination was noted. Catatonic features

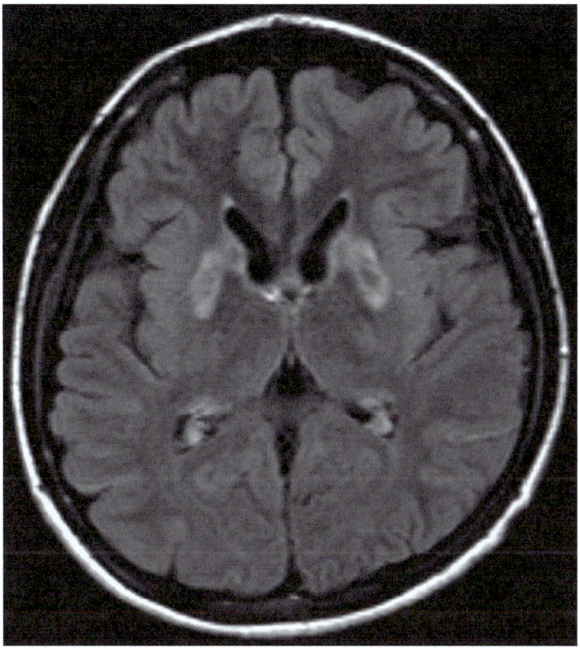

Fig. 27.1 Symmetrical T2 hyperintensity involving the corticospinal tracts bilaterally from the level of the posterior limb of the internal capsule extending inferiorly through the midbrain and into the pons

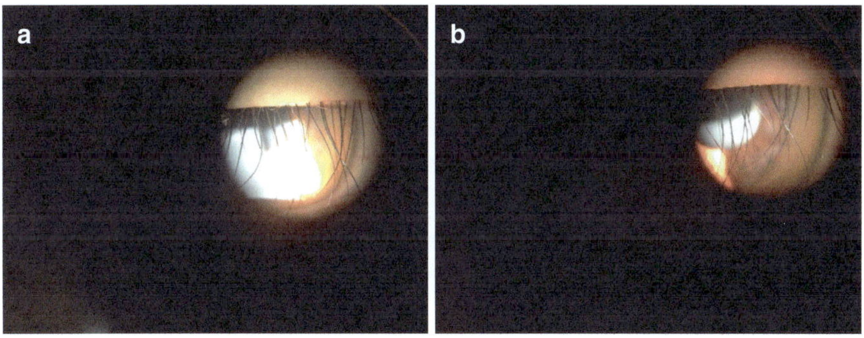

Fig. 27.2 (**a**, **b**) Kayser-Fleischer rings seen on ophthalmological examination

improved on trientine therapy, and lorazepam was not required. The autism symptoms were unchanged although his oppositional behaviors did improve.

What Did I Learn from This Case?

Adults with Wilson's disease often present with neuropsychiatric features [1], while children tend to present with liver disease [2]. However, children with Wilson's disease may present with unusual sudden-onset psychiatric or neurological features. Autism is a common diagnosis among school-age children, with one recent study estimating the prevalence to be between 11.3 and 15.6 per 1,000 [3]. In this case, the presence of autism complicated the picture and led to a delay in diagnosis; the emerging psychiatric symptoms were presumed to be due to the autism and so not extensively investigated. There were important clues in the history (nosebleeds, tremor, diarrhea) and abnormal liver function tests 2 years prior to diagnosis. The tremor exacerbated by penicillin therapy is interesting and should have alerted the clinicians to the possibility of Wilson's disease, as penicillin-type medications mobilize copper from the liver into the blood before excretion and can temporarily exacerbate neurological symptoms.

There are multiple etiologies in autism spectrum disorder, and genetic mechanisms are being increasingly described. It remains to be determined if children with Wilson's disease are at a higher risk of autism symptoms early in life. It is important to remember that autism features may coexist or be symptoms seen in associated conditions and may still need investigation especially if new symptoms emerge.

As neurometabolic conditions may be amenable to treatment, it is extremely important to recognize when a child with autism has atypical features (epilepsy, dysmorphic features, hypoglycemia, movement disorder) and warrants referral for further investigation [4, 5].

The final learning point and an important one clinically is that penicillamine treatment can trigger a worsening of neurological symptoms in Wilson's disease [6]. This occurs because penicillamine temporarily mobilizes large stores of copper from the liver into the blood and across the blood-brain barrier [6]. Trientine therapy is helpful in this context, as it is also a copper chelator and inhibits gut absorption of copper.

We thank Mr Amaya for providing the clinical photograph.

References

1. Brewer GJ. Neurologically presenting Wilson's disease: epidemiology, pathophysiology and treatment. CNS Drugs. 2005;19(3):185–92.
2. Ala A, et al. Wilson's disease. Lancet. 2007;369(9559):397–408.
3. Baron-Cohen S, et al. Prevalence of autism-spectrum conditions: UK school-based population study. Br J Psychiatry. 2009;194(6):500–9.
4. Gorker I, Tuzun U. Autistic-like findings associated with a urea cycle disorder in a 4-year-old girl. J Psychiatry Neurosci. 2005;30(2):133–5.
5. Manzi B, et al. Autism and metabolic diseases. J Child Neurol. 2008;23(3):307–14.
6. Brewer GJ, et al. Worsening of neurologic syndrome in patients with Wilson's disease with initial penicillamine therapy. Arch Neurol. 1987;44(5):490–3.

Chapter 28
With the Help of a German Dermatologist

Josef Priller

Admission

AP is a 42-year-old female who was admitted to our neuropsychiatric ward with a 2-month history of paranoid psychosis. She reported having lost control of her thoughts when her son unexpectedly arrived in Berlin. She had become increasingly irritable and experienced "unusual things." She started wandering around town barefoot and prayed. She claimed to have heard bomber planes arriving and helped to prevent the third world war with her prayers. She felt estranged with the country and left alone in a fight against all. Eventually, she attacked a pedestrian with a knife because she suspected him of being a radical who had bewitched his dog.

Background History

AP is reported to have been impulsive and irritable since her childhood. She developed a weakness for gambling in her youth but never came into conflict with the law. There is no history of substance abuse. She attended general school and now works in a restaurant. She is married and has a 16-year-old son. Allegedly, she has always been quite jealous and tries to steer her husband and son clear of others. At the age of 35, she developed renal insufficiency as a result of polycystic kidney disease. She required kidney transplantation and received a living donation from her husband. AP suffered two episodes of stroke, one pontomesencephalic stroke with transient diplopia and one right thalamic ischemic stroke. She was diagnosed with schizophrenia at the age of 40 after a first episode of paranoid psychosis with religious delusions.

J. Priller, MD
Department of Neuropsychiatry, Charité – Universitätsmedizin Berlin, Berlin, Germany
e-mail: josef.priller@charite.de

J. Priller, H. Rickards (eds.), *Neuropsychiatry Case Studies*,
DOI 10.1007/978-3-319-42190-2_28

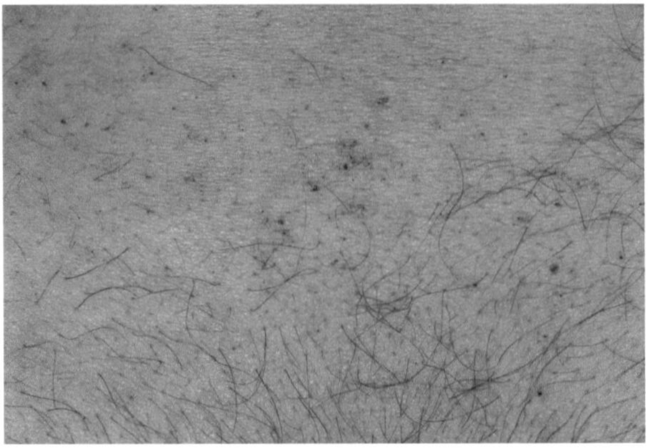

Fig. 28.1 Cluster of angiokeratomas

The productive symptoms remitted under risperidone treatment, but extrapyramidal side effects restricted dosing of the atypical antipsychotic drug to 2 mg per day. Medication adherence was low, and AP eventually discontinued her antipsychotic and immunosuppressive treatment.

Examination

She was alert and orientated. Attention and concentration were reduced and executive functions maintained. Her Mini-Mental State Examination score was 25. Thinking was slowed. She suffered from persecutory delusions and auditory hallucinations. Her affect was blunted. Neurological examination was normal with the exception of left-sided hyperreflexia. A reddish-purple rash was present in the groin (Fig. 28.1).

Initial Investigations

Routine blood screening revealed elevated levels of creatinine, myoglobin, C-reactive protein (CRP), and a mild anemia. Brain magnetic resonance imaging (MRI) showed old right thalamic and right pontine lacunar infarcts but no signs of leukoencephalopathy or blood-brain barrier disruption (Fig. 28.2).

Progress

We performed a lumbar puncture, which revealed a mild pleocytosis (41/μl, 84 % lymphocytes, 9 % monocytes, 7 % neutrophils), elevated protein level (835 mg/l), and normal lactate and glucose levels in the cerebrospinal fluid (CSF). IgG

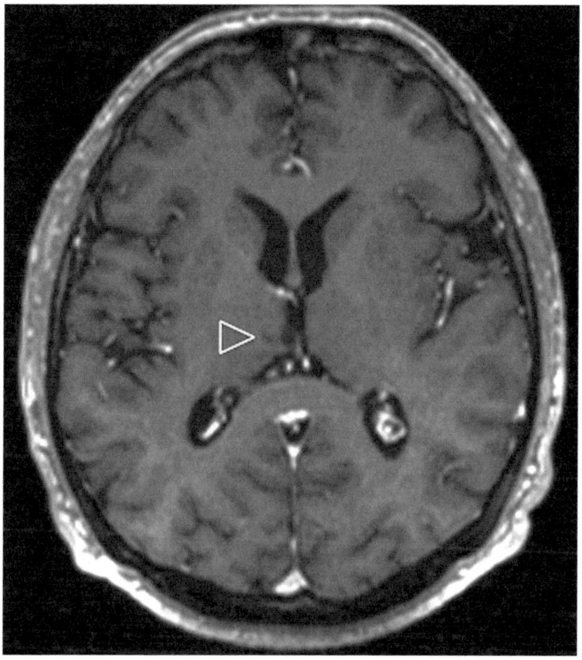

Fig. 28.2 Head MRI shows no gadolinium contrast enhancement in the T1-weighted sequences. The *arrowhead* indicates an old lacunar infarct in the right medial thalamus

oligoclonal bands unique to the CSF were detected. Viral encephalitis workup uncovered IgG antibodies specific to herpes simplex virus (HSV) 1 and 2, varicella-zoster virus (VZV), cytomegalovirus (CMV), and Epstein-Barr virus (EBV) in the serum and CSF. Polymerase chain reaction in the CSF was negative for HSV1, HSV2, VZV, CMV, and EBV deoxyribonucleic acids. Autoimmune screening revealed normal serum levels of antinuclear antibodies, circulating immune complexes, complement C3c and C4, and anticardiolipin antibodies. All coagulation parameters were normal. We suspected autoimmune encephalitis and sent blood and CSF samples to Angela Vincent at the University of Oxford. The autoantibody testing revealed anti-leucine-rich glioma-inactivated-1 (LGI1) antibodies in the CSF and serum.

Differential Diagnosis

The most obvious diagnosis in this case was organic psychosis. We found no evidence of rheumatoid arthritis, lupus, or other rheumatic diseases. The brain MRI findings without signs of demyelination were not suggestive of multiple sclerosis. Instead, the patient's family history of polycystic kidney disease (mother, uncle, and aunt), arterial hypertension and cardiac disease (father and brother), diabetes, and stroke (brother) suggested Fabry's disease (Anderson-Fabry disease), a rare X-linked inborn error of metabolism [1]. The diagnosis was confirmed by our dermatologists, who performed a skin biopsy and found lysosomal lipid deposits in endothelial cells of angiokeratomas and reduced α-galactosidase A activity in skin fibroblasts. Ophthalmological assessment of AP revealed corneal opacities (cornea verticillata), a typical ocular sign of Fabry's disease. We also detected severe cardiac disease with concentric left (and right) ventricular hypertrophy and mitral insufficiency, but no shunt. Carotid and transcranial Doppler ultrasound were normal.

Further Investigation

The presence of CSF-specific oligoclonal bands and a mild lymphocytic pleocytosis, as well as increased serum CRP, indicated an immune response in AP. Interestingly, chronic meningitis and lacunar strokes have previously been described in two young females with Fabry's disease [2, 3]. Testing for infectious agents or serum autoantibodies was negative. Our screening for disease-relevant autoantibodies revealed serum and CSF antibodies to LGI1, a member of the Kv1 voltage-gated potassium channel complex (VGKC). LGI1 antibodies were first described in patients with limbic encephalitis or epilepsy, all without tumors [4, 5]. Notably, VGKC autoimmunity has been associated with frequent psychiatric manifestations; psychotic symptoms such as hallucinations and delusions occur in more than 20 % of cases [6, 7].

Diagnosis

The diagnosis of autoimmune encephalitis with VGKC complex LGI1 antibodies in a patient with Fabry's disease was made. She was treated successfully with immunosuppression (mycophenolate mofetil and tacrolimus), antipsychotics (risperidone long-acting injections), and enzyme replacement therapy (agalsidase alfa).

What Did I Learn from This Case?

I learned that it is important to fully examine the patient, including the skin, which provided an important diagnostic cue in this case. The German dermatologist Johannes Fabry first described the characteristic angiokeratoma in what was later to be called Fabry's disease [8] or Anderson-Fabry disease in recognition of the English surgeon, William Anderson, who independently described the disease. I also learned that heterozygous females are not asymptomatic carriers of the X-linked lysosomal storage disorder as previously assumed, but the majority develop Fabry's disease with typical organ involvement (Fig. 28.3), including a high risk of cardiac disease and stroke [1, 9, 10].

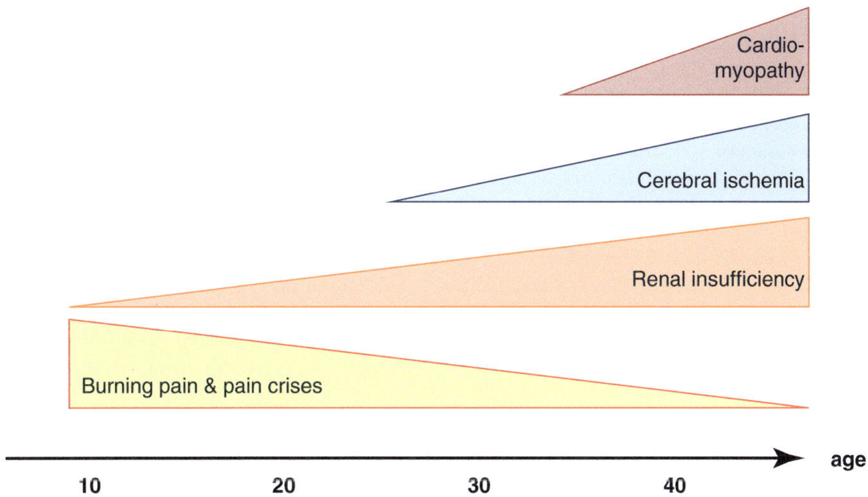

Fig. 28.3 Different clinical manifestations in Fabry's disease (mod. from [18])

Finally, I learned that psychiatric symptoms are common in Fabry's disease. In fact, 50–60% of individuals with Fabry's disease suffer from depression [11, 12]. Psychosis has also been reported in Fabry's disease, but was mostly diagnosed as concurrent schizophrenia [13, 14]. Interestingly, thalamic lesions have been implicated in the pathogenesis of psychotic symptoms in another patient with Fabry's disease, who also demonstrated increased sensitivity to the extrapyramidal side effects of risperidone [15].

Notably, this is the first case of Fabry's disease associated with autoimmune encephalopathy. It should be pointed out that a high incidence of autoantibodies (against extractable nuclear antigens, cardiolipin, and phospholipid) has been detected in Fabry's disease [16]. Moreover, Fabry's disease can be preceded by autoimmune hypothyroidism [17], suggesting potential elements of overlap.

Bibliography

1. Zarate YA, Hopkin RJ. Fabry's disease. Lancet. 2008;372:1427–35.
2. Schreiber W, Udvardi A, Kristoferitsch W. Chronic meningitis and lacunar stroke in Fabry disease. J Neurol. 2007;254:1447–9.
3. Lidove O, Chauveheid M-P, Benoist L, Alexandra J-F, Klein I, Papo T. Chronic meningitis and thalamic involvement in a woman: Fabry disease expanding phenotype. J Neurol Neurosurg Psychiatry. 2007;78:1007–13.
4. Lai M, Huijbers MG, Lancaster E, Graus F, Bataller L, Balice-Gordon R, Cowell JK, Dalmau J. Investigation of LGI1 as the antigen in limbic encephalitis previously attributed to potassium channels: a case series. Lancet Neurol. 2010;9:776–85.
5. Irani SR, Alexander S, Waters P, Kleopa KA, Pettingill P, Zuliani L, Peles E, Buckley C, Lang B, Vincent A. Antibodies to Kv1 potassium channel-complex proteins leucine-rich, glioma

inactivated 1 protein and contactin-associated protein-2 in limbic encephalitis, Morvan's syndrome and acquired neuromyotonia. Brain. 2010;133:2734–48.
6. Somers KJ, Lennon VA, Rundell JR, Pittock SJ, Drubach DA, Trenerry MR, Lachance DH, Klein CJ, Aston PA, McKeon A. Psychiatric manifestations of voltage-gated potassium-channel complex autoimmunity. J Neuropsychiatry Clin Neurosci. 2011;23:425–33.
7. Parthasarathi UD, Harrower T, Tempest M, Hodges JR, Walsh C, McKenna PJ, Fletcher PC. Psychiatric presentation of voltage-gated potassium channel antibody-associated encephalopathy. Case report. Br J Psychiatry. 2006;189:182–3.
8. Fabry J. Ein Beitrag zur Kenntnis der Purpura haemorrhagica nodularis (Purpura papulosa haemorrhagica Hebrae). Arch Dermatol Syph. 1898;43:187–200.
9. Wilcox WR, Oliveira JP, Hopkin RJ, Ortiz A, Banikazemi M, Feldt-Rasmussen U, Sims K, Waldek S, Pastores GM, Lee P, Eng CM, Marodi L, Stanford KE, Breunig F, Wanner C, Warnock DG, Lemay RM, Germain DP, Registry F. Females with Fabry disease frequently have major organ involvement: lessons from the Fabry registry. Mol Genet Metab. 2008;93:112–28.
10. Fellgiebel A, Müller MJ, Ginsberg L. CNS manifestations of Fabry's disease. Lancet Neurol. 2006;5:791–5.
11. Cole AL, Lee PJ, Hughes DA, Deegan PB, Waldek S, Lachmann RH. Depression in adults with Fabry disease: a common and under-diagnosed problem. J Inherit Metab Dis. 2007;30:943–51.
12. Lelieveld IM, Böttcher A, Hennermann JB, Beck M, Fellgiebel A. Eight-year follow-up of neuropsychiatric symptoms and brain structural changes in Fabry disease. PLoS ONE. 2015;10:e0137603.
13. Liston EH, Levine MD, Philippart M. Psychosis in Fabry disease and treatment with phenoxybenzamine. Arch Gen Psychiatry. 1973;29:402–3.
14. Gairing S, Wiest R, Metzler S, Theodoridou A, Hoff P. Fabry's disease and psychosis: causality or coincidence? Psychopathology. 2011;44:201–4.
15. Shen YC, Haw-Ming L, Lin CC, Chen CH. Psychosis in a patient with Fabry's disease and treatment with aripiprazole. Prog Neuropsychopharmacol Biol Psychiatry. 2007;31:779–80.
16. Martinez P, Aggio M, Rozenfeld P. High incidence of autoantibodies in Fabry disease patients. J Inherit Metab Dis. 2007;30:365–9.
17. Katsumata N, Ishiguro A, Watanabe H. Fabry disease superimposed on overt autoimmune hypothyroidism. Clin Pediatr Endocrinol. 2011;20:95–8.
18. Goldsmith LA, Katz SI, Gilchrest BA, Paller AS, Leffell DJ, Wolff K. Fitzpatricks's Dermatology in General Medicine, 8th Edn.: www.accessmedicine.com.

Chapter 29
A Musician Presents with Unusual Facial Movements, Insomnia, and Depression

Mark Groves

Presenting History

RB, a relatively healthy 68-year-old musician, is referred for psychiatric treatment after reporting several months of distressing episodic movements. His partner described the sudden-onset episodes as spasm-like flexing of one arm and hand, accompanied by bizarre facial grimaces. The episodes, which occurred day and night and lasted 1–2 s, had been increasing in frequency over the few months prior to evaluation. Nocturnal episodes could approach 45 per night, severely disrupting his sleep. Episodes were associated with speech arrest but preserved consciousness and "weird, intrusive thoughts and images," such as thinking of the letter "X."

Examinations

During the initial consultations with a movement disorder neurologist, examinations were completely normal. His doctor observed a few brief episodic movements described as dystonic or myoclonic because of their variable quality. Due to insomnia, RB was referred to a sleep specialist who observed the movements and was concerned they might be partial seizures. She recommended further testing and evaluation by a general neurologist. The neurological workup was normal despite observed movement episodes that, based on their appearance, were considered unlikely to be seizures. Multiple tests were ordered to thoroughly rule out seizures or other diagnoses.

M. Groves, MD
Department of Psychiatry, Icahn School of Medicine at Mt. Sinai, New York, NY, USA
e-mail: mgroves@chpnet.org

J. Priller, H. Rickards (eds.), *Neuropsychiatry Case Studies*,
DOI 10.1007/978-3-319-42190-2_29

Initial Investigations

Routine blood screening, comprehensive metabolic panel, and TSH were all normal. Antiphospholipid antibodies, ANA, anti-dsDNA, lupus anticoagulant, Lyme studies, and ceruloplasmin were negative. A paraneoplastic panel was pending though clinical suspicion was low for an occult malignancy.

MRI of the brain and cervical spine was clinically insignificant and 24-h video EEG normal and without electrographic correlate. Given these results, RB's episodes were suspected to be of non-epileptic origin. A sleep study indicated severely fragmented sleep, no observed REM sleep, and no evidence of epileptiform activity or sleep-disordered breathing.

Differential Diagnosis

Initial diagnostic considerations included partial seizures, a movement disorder such as myoclonus-dystonia, a complex sleep disorder possibly due to escalating hypnic-myoclonic jerks, and functional movements accompanied by depression and anxiety. Given the strange phenomenology – apparent distractibility, suggestibility, and high variability of the episodes along with negative EEG – seizures and myoclonus-dystonia were thought to be highly unlikely.

Initial Treatment and Psychiatric Referral

Clonazepam was prescribed and gradually increased, with little reported benefit. RB was thought to have depressive symptoms and decreased motivation, energy, and concentration, so escitalopram was prescribed along with a referral for psychiatric evaluation and treatment. The history was reviewed at intake, and RB could not identify any clear precipitating stressor at movement onset but acknowledged some depressive symptoms, decreased motivation, fatigue, and memory and cognitive changes. He was uncertain how much the cognitive changes were related to his sleep difficulties. His partner reported, "He is not the man I knew."

RB was open to the possibility of a functional diagnosis and had been trying to find any links to thought content that seemed to precipitate movements. He was very attentive to when he would have movements, especially at night, which seemed to compound his insomnia. He had started to keep logs and count the number of episodes; it seemed his guardedness and anxious anticipation of movements facilitated their escalation.

Past psychiatric and psychosocial history was unremarkable. Family psychiatric history was notable for bipolar disorder in his father. Family neurological history was negative, although his sister had a mild autoimmune thyroid disorder.

During the interview, he was observed to have a few episodes of facial grimacing and arm flexion with fanning of the fingers – the phenomenology varied from episode to episode and was very strange appearing. Episodes could be interrupted by distraction and seemed to become more frequent during discussion of life stressors or the movements themselves.

Clinical Course

On repeat laboratory testing soon after the psychiatric evaluation, he was found to be hyponatremic with an Na of 121. The hyponatremia was suspected to be due to SIADH secondary to the escitalopram, so it was discontinued. The plan was to wait until normalization of the Na and then consider an alternative like Trazodone.

When the SIADH did not resolve despite SSRI discontinuation, RB was referred to a nephrologist. With fluid restriction, his Na approached normal. Trazodone, a non-SSRI antidepressant, was started to target the sleep disorder, depression, and hypervigilance that appeared to be exacerbating his symptoms. RB agreed to adhere to fluid restriction, while we closely monitored his Na. He reported some periods of sleeping well and occasional weeks with few symptoms, followed by a recurrence of symptoms and poor sleep the following week. He was encouraged by seemingly partial benefit, but movements continued, and his Na continued to fluctuate when he was not strictly adhering to fluid restriction. The nephrologist did not feel further workup was indicated.

RB and his partner subsequently reported a number of serious falls, one in particular causing severe bruising and a torn thigh muscle. In mid-January 2013, due to continued hyponatremia and concern for further risk of falls, the patient was admitted to the hospital for additional workup and treatment of persistent hyponatremia.

New Diagnosis

Upon admission, a thorough review by the medical and neurology teams revealed a moderately abnormal VGKC antibody level of 0.30 nmol/L (normal <0.02 nmol/L) in the paraneoplastic autoantibody panel that had previously been missed or considered clinically insignificant. Further antibody studies were completed, and the patient was subsequently diagnosed with faciobrachial dystonic seizures due to Lgi1 antibodies. Imaging of his whole body ruled out any occult malignancies, and a 5-day course of IV steroid therapy resulted in notable benefit. He felt cognitively clearer, his Na improved, and his movements abated. The patient continued to improve at home. By late February, his Na had normalized, he was feeling significantly better, and he began monthly IVIG therapy. A second course of IV steroids was administered a few months later, after a slight recurrence of nighttime movements. RB seemed to have a better response to IV steroids, so the IVIG therapy was discontinued. With continued monthly treatments and close monitoring of Lgi1-Abs, the patient remains stable and has been able to resume work and his musical performances.

Case Learning Points

This has been one of the most instructive cases of my career. I learned that autoimmune channelopathies are a new and important area to consider yet are too often dismissed as functional conditions. The bizarre and fluctuating phenomenology in RB's case was perplexing and confused the picture: was the insomnia caused by hypnic jerks? Did its severity explain the cognitive complaints, thought disorder, fatigue, and movements? Was SIADH secondary to SSRI therapy? In retrospect, one underlying neurological process could more parsimoniously explain the full constellation of symptoms. Furthermore, there had been recently published cases in the literature with remarkably similar semiology.

This case highlights the importance of developing a high index of suspicion for these recently described channelopathies, which are responsive to immunotherapy especially when started early in the clinical course. There should be a low threshold for performing fully up-to-date autoimmune screening panels. The mildly abnormal VGKC-Abs level was retested, and more specific antibody analyses confirmed Lgi1-specific antibodies.

The knowledge base of neuropsychiatry is ever evolving – it requires conscientious literature review to keep up with new developments. Over time, it is highly likely that a subset of patients referred to psychiatry for functional disorders will be re-diagnosed with more specific conditions akin to this autoimmune channelopathy, resulting in more specific and effective treatments.

Key Points

- Autoimmune channelopathies are a new and important area to consider.
- Often misdiagnosed as functional conditions.
- Manifest as a range of neurological symptoms involving different areas of the nervous system.
- Should be considered in the presence of sudden-onset seizures particularly when associated with neuropsychiatric features and cognitive disturbances.
- Are clinically responsive to immunotherapy treatments.

Chapter 30
The Division Between Psychiatric and Neurological Practice Does Not Help Patients with Disorders That Span the Two

Belinda Lennox

IT was a 19-year-old student who presented to the psychiatric services during his first term at University with a 1-month history of altered mental state. His main difficulties were with sleep, poor concentration, low mood, and paranoid psychosis. His sleep complaint was of hypersomnia. Undisturbed he would sleep for up to 18 h each day. When he forced himself to wake up for lectures, he would then find himself irresistibly sleepy during the day. When awake he found that his concentration and attention were very poor and he was unable to retain any information that was relayed in tutorials. His mood had deteriorated such that he got no enjoyment from social events, which he had previously looked forward to. He felt hopeless about his situation and had some thoughts that he might be better off dead and was contemplating suicide. His appetite was reduced and he had lost some weight. He had also developed paranoid thoughts that others were watching him, perhaps monitoring him through CCTV cameras, although he wasn't 100 % convinced about this, and he was hearing whispering voices talking to him, although he couldn't make out what they were saying.

Of relevance in his past he was a high-achieving, hardworking student who had received previous treatment with SSRIs for anxiety around the time of his school exams that was attributed to the particular stress at that time. He had no other medical history, and there was no family history of mental illness. He did not drink or take any illicit drugs.

The initial differential diagnosis was either of an atypical depressive disorder or an evolving first-episode psychosis. He was treated with SSRI antidepressants and a low-dose second-generation antipsychotic, and he was followed up by the community mental health team. Routine blood screening did not show any abnormalities.

B. Lennox, BMedSci, BM, BS, MRCPsych
Department of Psychiatry, University of Oxford, Warneford Hospital, Headington, Oxford, UK
e-mail: belinda.lennox@psych.ox.ac.uk

J. Priller, H. Rickards (eds.), *Neuropsychiatry Case Studies*,
DOI 10.1007/978-3-319-42190-2_30

Unfortunately over the next few months, his symptoms worsened, such that he was sleeping for up to 20 h a day and unable to take part in any academic work at all. When awake, he had intense thoughts and images of himself committing suicide, by jumping off a bridge in particular. His paranoid ideas were now fixed, such that he was convinced that he was being monitored and that he may be part of a large conspiracy. His antidepressant and antipsychotic treatments were increased and then changed, but with no benefit. He received intensive support at home, with daily visits from the community mental health team.

At this point his serum was tested for antineuronal cell surface antibodies and tested positive for anti-NMDAR antibodies at a level of 1:50. He was given further investigation and had a normal EEG, MRI, CSF, and paraneoplastic screen.

He was treated with a course of plasma exchange and 3 days of methylprednisolone 500 mg orally. He reported an improvement of his sleep and psychosis within 2 weeks of plasma exchange and he was able to resume his university course within the month.

What Did I Learn from This Case?

I learned a number of lessons from this case. My professional background as a psychiatrist has biased me toward making psychiatric diagnoses in patients presenting with neuropsychiatric symptoms. The level of hypersomnia described by this patient was extreme and should have alerted me earlier to an organic process. In fact, it was so extreme that the response from some of the mental health team was that they didn't believe him. Historically, unfortunately, this has often been the response to patients when they present with symptoms that don't fit in with our previous clinical experience. I also learned that although the level of the antibodies was relatively low in this patient, and he didn't have other features of an encephalopathy, he still made a significant, temporally related, improvement in his mental state following immunotherapy that he had not had with several months of psychiatric treatment. It is therefore likely that the antibodies were relevant to the clinical syndrome in this patient.

Differential Diagnosis of Hypersomnia

Hypothalamic tumors
Kleine-Levin syndrome
Endocrine/metabolic causes – hypothyroidism
Encephalitis lethargica
Narcolepsy
Other forms of paraneoplastic limbic encephalitis

Bibliography

1. Dalmau J, Lancaster E, Martinez-Hernandez E, Rosenfeld MR, Balice-Gordon R. Clinical experience and laboratory investigations in patients with anti-NMDAR encephalitis. Lancet Neurol. 2011;10:63–74.
2. Irani SR, Bera K, Waters P, Zuliani L, Maxwell S, Zandi MS, Friese MA, Galea I, Kullmann DM, Beeson D, Lang B, Bien CG, Vincent A. N-methyl-D-aspartate antibody encephalitis: temporal progression of clinical and paraclinical observations in a predominantly non-paraneoplastic disorder of both sexes. Brain. 2010;133:1655–67.
3. Vincent A, Bien CG, Irani SR, Waters P. Autoantibodies associated with diseases of the CNS: new developments and future challenges. Lancet Neurol. 2011;10:759–72.
4. Zandi MS, Deakin JB, Coles AJ, Cox A, Jones PB, Vincent A, Lennox BR. Immunotherapy for patients with acute psychosis and serum N-methyl D-aspartate receptor (NMDAR) antibodies: a description of a treated case series. Schizophr Res. 2014;160:193–5.

Chapter 31
First-Episode Psychosis with Autoimmune Antibodies Involving Clear Neuropsychological Impairment with Common and Unusual Features

Patrick Vesey, Paul Maddison, Eileen Ellen T. O'Regan, and Eleanor Williams

Summary

Encephalitis is an acute inflammatory condition of the brain caused by infective or autoimmune mechanisms. It typically involves headache, fever, confusion, seizures, and sensory or motor disturbance. Recently there have been increased understandings of the role of neuronal cell antibodies in presentations of encephalitis that have psychiatric features only.

Presentation

DL presented as a 32-year-old male manual worker in May 2014 with sudden-onset psychosis involving paranoid persecutory delusions and auditory hallucinations, without infective prodrome. He referred to his mind feeling muddled and confused. His mood was low but he had insight (which he retained throughout). He was admitted to inpatient psychiatric care. He was otherwise well. He lived with his wife and children. He smoked cigarettes and took alcohol in moderation. He denied illicit drug use. There was no family psychiatric history. He was initially commenced on quetiapine XL to a maximum dose of 400 mg which was discontinued due to

P. Vesey, BSc (Hons), D Clin Psych (✉) • E. Williams, BSc, MSc
Department of Clinical Psychology and Neuropsychology,
Nottingham University Hospitals NHS Trust, Queen's Medical Centre,
Nottingham, UK
e-mail: Patrick.Vesey@nuh.nhs.uk; patrick.vesey@nhs.net

P. Maddison, MD, FRCP
Department of Neurology, Queen's Medical Centre, Nottingham, UK

E.E.T. O'Regan, MB, BCh, BAO, MRCPsych
Marlow House, Early Intervention in Psychosis Service, Nottingham, UK
e-mail: eleanor.williams3@nuh.nhs.uk

J. Priller, H. Rickards (eds.), *Neuropsychiatry Case Studies*,
DOI 10.1007/978-3-319-42190-2_31

tachycardia. That was then changed to aripiprazole to a maximum of 30 mg but with limited benefit, which was then changed to olanzapine up to a maximum of 20 mg.

Examination

Initial examination showed moderate cognitive impairment even against the background of limited educational background. Speech, vision, and swallowing were normal. He had no headaches. His weight was slightly reduced. He reported poor concentration and difficulty sleeping.

Initial Investigations

In July 2014, blood antibody screening was negative for NMDAR but slightly raised for anti-VGKC (361 pmol). He was referred for a neurology outpatient review, also remaining under the care of the early intervention in psychosis team. In October 2014, a second blood sample was confirmed as strongly positive having increased from the previous level (529 pmol). Pending neurology review, he was referred for CT imaging of the chest, abdomen, and pelvis.

Progress

At his first outpatient neurology review in December 2014, the previous history was confirmed. His psychosis remained prominent. On examination, there was no ataxia. He had slight twitches in his fingers but no fasciculation elsewhere. Fundoscopy was normal with visible venous pulsations bilaterally. The rest of the cranial nerves were entirely normal. Muscle, tone, power, and reflexes were normal throughout with flexor plantar responses. Light touch sensation was normal. There was no pseudomyotonia. His hands became a little tremulous but without muscle rippling or cramps, and he had no abnormal facial movements. He wondered whether his gait had been unsteady, but he had no skin rash or difficulties with handgrip release. Sphincteric function was normal. There was no history or family history of autoimmunity.

Differential Diagnosis

It was felt that apart from the minor finger twitching in the hands, he did not have any of the usual features of patients with potassium channel antibodies, such as peripheral nerve hyperexcitability or encephalitis, and the neurological management options were therefore felt to be uncertain. However it was felt that immunosuppression was an option and advice was sought on what treatment regimens might be helpful.

Investigation and Management

Potassium channel antibody levels were found to be increased (782 pmol). Brain MRI with and without gadolinium was reported as normal (November 2014). EMG was reported as normal (December 2014). EEG was also reported as normal (January 2015). CT chest showed a small mass, possibly a thymoma (February 2015).

His psychotic symptoms remained prominent despite ongoing review and increase of his medication (olanzapine to 20 mg, February 2015). In view of the ongoing marked psychosis, it was agreed that he would have a neurology admission for a 5-day course of intravenous immunoglobulin.

He underwent 5-day intravenous immunoglobulin (40 g per day for 5 days, February 2015). At the start, his Addenbrooke's ACE-R was 45/100 (attention 9/18, memory 6/26, fluency 1/14, language 16/26, visuospatial 13/16). Toward the end, his Addenbrooke's was 52/100 (attention 11/18, memory 10/26, fluency 3/14, language 15/26, visuospatial 13/16). This was regarded as a minor nominal increase in his Addenbrooke's results, of uncertain clinical significance.

Following IVIG treatment, he was commenced on prednisolone although the dose was limited due to liver function abnormalities. He reported perhaps slightly reduced hallucinations.

More detailed outpatient neuropsychology was commenced (April 2015) but was limited by the difficulty he experienced in attempting the procedures. Brief results were yielded. On a test of remote semantic memory (WAIS III [1] Information, a general knowledge test), a low result was obtained (SS 4); it was unclear whether this denoted loss of general knowledge as a result of his illness or whether it reflected poor long-term knowledge perhaps as a result of limited formal education.

Notably on a figure-copy test, a markedly abnormal performance was evident involving stark counterclockwise reproduction of the figure. In view of the possibility of DL having misunderstood the requirement of the procedure, he was asked to draw the figure again but again produced a counterclockwise-oriented drawing of the figure. DL's rotated drawings are shown in Figs. 31.1 and 31.2.

Rotated drawings in neuropsychological assessments are a rare abnormal finding, if somewhat nonspecific [2]. They are traditionally regarded as having an unequivocal organic basis. Object perception, naming, and recognition are usually intact in patients who produce a grossly rotated drawing; such distortions can occur even for line drawings of common objects which are correctly named. Occipitoparietal processes (dorsal stream) are implicated. Rotational errors have previously been reported in cases of psychosis and schizophrenia but sometimes to only a small

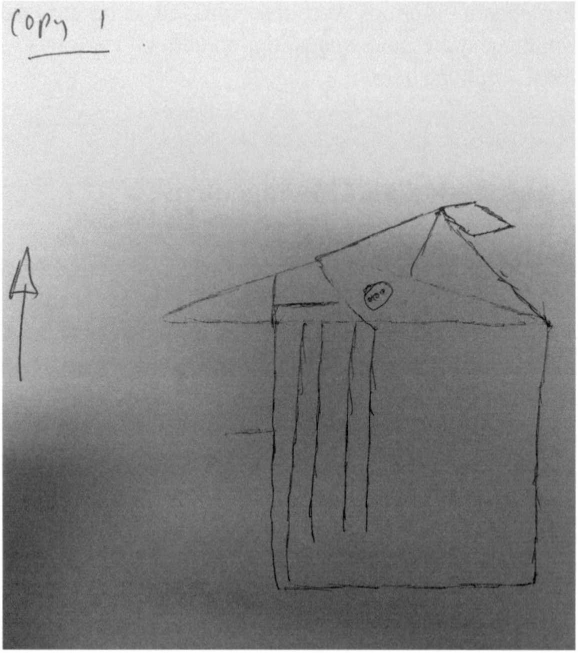

Fig. 31.1 Patient's counterclockwise drawings

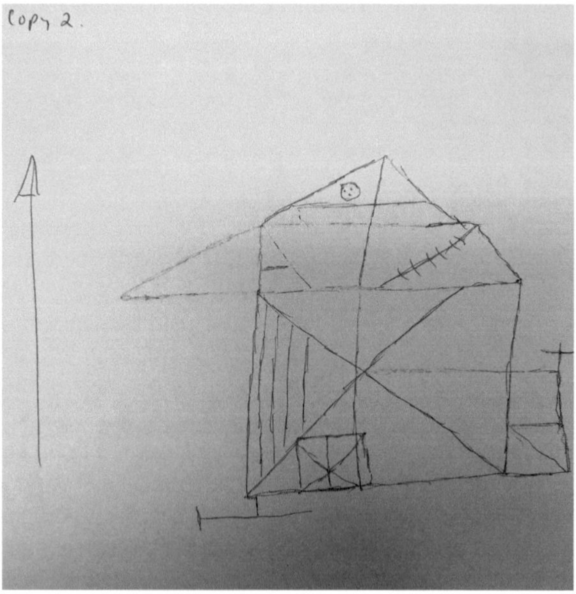

Fig. 31.2 Patient's counterclockwise drawings

degree and less so than other drawing-copy errors [3]. Subtle but distinct perceptual disturbance has also been reported in cases of autoimmune encephalitis presenting neuropsychiatrically [4].

Progress and Diagnosis

Close liaison continued between the relevant services, but unfortunately his attendance was sometimes patchy particularly for neurology outpatients and related investigations. There were concerns about his concordance, related to being forgetful, and he had a depot trial of pipothiazine palmitate in June 2015, which was discontinued because of extrapyramidal side effects. By November 2015, his repeat anti-VGKC levels were much lower, almost normal at 210 pmol. However his psychosis remained troubling for him. His medication included olanzapine 20 mg and mirtazapine 15 mg, and he was considering a trial of clozapine but had so far been unable to watch an informational DVD about it. He was attending hearing voices workshops and doing more therapeutic activities. His chest mass was not thought to be sinister, on MDT review, but remained under surveillance.

At the time of writing, investigations and multidisciplinary management of the case are ongoing. The earlier putative formulation of the case as one of autoimmune encephalitis presenting as first-episode psychosis has been subject to reconsideration, largely in view of the limited responsiveness of the psychosis to the immunotherapy.

What Have We Learned from This Case?

(a) This case of first-episode psychosis with raised autoimmune antibodies raises the question of the significance of neuronal cell antibodies in the patient's presentation. Management is ongoing.
(b) There are marked cognitive and neuropsychological signs; some are clinically common, while others, involving apparent perceptual disturbance, are very unusual.
(c) It invites further study of the prevalence of such neuropsychological signs in similar cases.
(d) The case reinforces recent cross-discipline advances in the understanding of psychosis/schizophrenia: specifically, that presentations of psychosis exist that involve distinctly abnormal neurology.
(e) The case also reinforces the complexities that can be involved in managing such conditions, where patient engagement can be variable or poor, from the perspective of highly specialist services located in different healthcare settings.

References

1. Wechsler adult intelligence scale – 3rd Edition. Psychological Corporation; 1997.
2. Solms, et al. Rotated drawing: the range of performance and anatomical correlates in a series of 16 patients. Brain Cogn. 1998;38:358–68.
3. Dridan BA, Ong B, Lloyd S, Evans L, Crowe SF. The simple copy task: detecting higher order visual processing deficits in schizophrenia, dementia, and movement disorder groups. Aust Psychol. 2013;48(2):98–109.
4. Eg. As reported in Cahalan, S. Brain on fire: my month of madness. Penguin; 2013.

Chapter 32
Subacute Onset of Psychosis with Epileptic Seizures and Dysautonomia: Think Autoimmunity!

Til Menge, Diamandis Toutzaris, and Rüdiger J. Seitz

RG is a 23-year-old, previously healthy woman who recently completed her training to become a tracer. Eight weeks prior to her admission to our institution, she experienced a series of generalized epileptic fits over a period of 5 days. Neurological examination and an extensive diagnostic workup, including cranial MR imaging (MRI) and lumbar puncture (LP), were unremarkable. Due to ongoing agitation and delusions, she had to be transferred to a secure psychiatric ward where she continued to experience epileptic fits and also episodes of fainting. After an interdisciplinary neurological psychiatric discussion, blood tests for anti-NMDA-NR1 antibodies were ordered and returned positive twice for serum IgG (titer 1:100 and 1:320, respectively) 7 weeks after onset and 6 weeks after psychiatric admission. A follow-up MRI revealed subtle T2 hyperintensities compatible with limbic encephalitis. On a repeat LP anti-NMDA-NR1, antibodies were also detected in the otherwise completely normal cerebrospinal fluid (CSF; 1:10; normal <1:2). The electroencephalogram (EEG) showed generalized slowing without epileptic discharge patterns (Fig. 32.1). An ovarian teratoma was ruled out by repeated gynecological examinations and by pelvic MRI. The patient was treated with 5 days of intravenous (i.v.) high-dose methylprednisolone (IVMP) followed by 5 days of i.v. immunoglobulins (IVIg, total of 100 g). Her condition improved steadily, and she was referred to a neuro-rehabilitation unit 4 weeks later. Also, an autonomic dysfunction was diagnosed by means of a pathological sympathetic skin reaction (SSR), which reverted to normal prior to discharge, concomitant with the cessation of faints. On follow-up 7 months later, she was near normal with only subtle mnestic abnormalities as assessed by neuropsychological testing, but there were no psychosis, further fits, or faints. Importantly, she was off any antipsychotic or anticonvulsive medication.

T. Menge, MD • D. Toutzaris, MD • R.J. Seitz, MD (✉)
Department of Neurology, LVR-Klinikum Düsseldorf, Heinrich-Heine-University Düsseldorf, Düsseldorf, Germany
e-mail: til.menge@lvr.de; toutzari@uni-duesseldorf.de; seitz@neurologie.uni-duesseldorf.de

J. Priller, H. Rickards (eds.), *Neuropsychiatry Case Studies*,
DOI 10.1007/978-3-319-42190-2_32

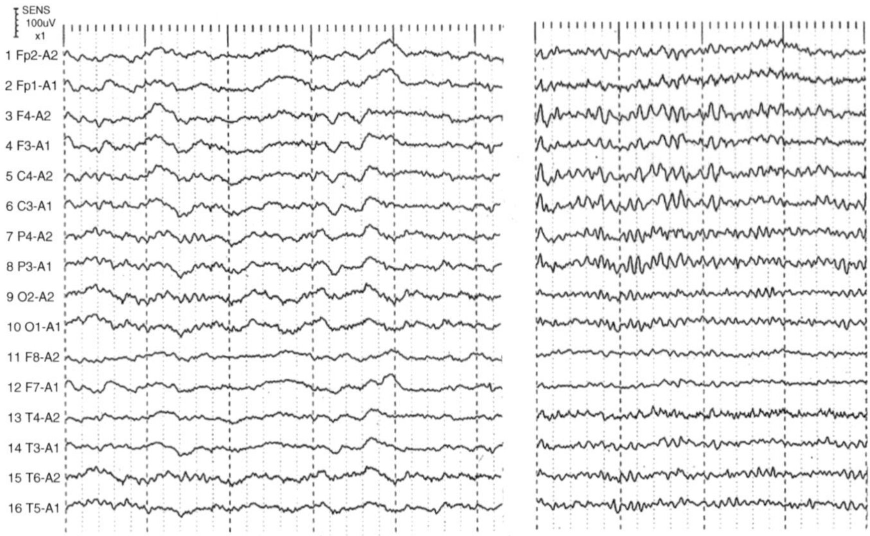

Fig. 32.1 Electroencephalograms of patient RG. *Left*: EEG during peak of disease showing generalized slowing. *Right*: EEG recorded 7.5 months later during remission showing normalized alpha activity

The second case (SB) is a 38-year-old male social pedagogue who experienced encephalitis and epileptic seizures 10 years ago. After an asymptomatic period, seizures reoccurred, followed by several panic attacks, sleeping disorder, brooding, and lack of concentration. These disturbances led the patient to seek consultancy from a psychiatric clinic, where depression was diagnosed and he was hospitalized. Due to his epileptic seizures, he was then referred to our center for a differential workup. The MRI showed no abnormality apart from a previously diagnosed volume decrease of his left temporal lobe. The EEG was normal, while his CSF revealed an elevated total protein (629 mg/L; normal: 150–450) and a raised albumin quotient indicative of a disrupted blood-brain barrier. During his stay on our ward, the patient experienced progressive delusions and sexual disinhibition and, thus, had to be transferred to a secure psychiatric ward. As soon as the presence of anti-NMDA-NR1 IgG antibodies both (1:32) in serum and CSF were detected, the patient was treated with IVMP over 5 days of IVMP followed by 5 days of IVIg, with a total of 120 g. A profound improvement of his psychopathological symptoms occurred after 4 weeks of neuropsychiatric rehabilitation.

Diagnosis

In both patients, the diagnosis of anti-NMDAR encephalitis was confirmed by the presence of serum and CSF antibodies against the N-methyl-D-aspartate receptor. These antibodies bind to the NR1 subunit, one of two subunits of the heterotetrameric receptor. Pathophysiologically, these antibodies suppress neuronal activity in vitro and reduce cell surface receptor densities in dissociated hippocampal neuron cultures [1, 2]. NMDARs are glutamate-gated ion channels that are expressed in the mammalian brain in abundance and are pivotal in regulating synapse function. In 2007, a novel paraneoplastic syndrome was described by Dalmau et al. [3]; the authors observed the presence of IgG autoantibodies directed against the NMDAR NR1/NR2 subunits in 12 female patients with ovarian teratoma, associated with clinical signs of psychosis, memory deficits, seizures, dyskinesia, decreased consciousness, and autonomic instability to a highly variable degree. Since then, more than 570 patients have been described [4]. In general, patients develop prominent psychiatric manifestations (acute behavioral change, psychosis, catatonia) that evolve to include seizures, memory deficits, extrapyramidal movement disorders (mainly dyskinesias), speech problems, and autonomic and ventilatory dysregulation to various extents. However, in a small proportion (approximately 4 %), the disease may manifest with isolated psychiatric symptoms [5]. Treatment of choice beyond symptomatic antipsychotic medication is anti-inflammatory. At the time of clinical suspicion or serological evidence, IVMP should be initiated. This should be followed by IVIg or plasmapheresis (PE). If remission, albeit slow, cannot be achieved or maintained, more aggressive second-line immunotherapies should be propagated, i.e., rituximab or cyclophosphamide. Importantly, an extensive search for an underlying malignancy has to be conducted to segregate a paraneoplastic (paraimmune) from a primary autoimmune anti-NMDAR encephalitis [4].

What Have We Learned from These Cases?

This series of two cases has taught us four key points.

- First, the anti-NMDAR encephalitis is all but rare and affects both sexes. All cases have been diagnosed and treated at our center within 1 year. Moreover, it appears that the proportion of anti-NMDAR encephalitis cases surpasses that of any specific viral cause in young individuals, probably not only in California [6].
- Second, the clinical presentation can be very variable, and subtle neurological, ictal, or dysautonomic signs may be masked by overt psychotic features that may result in an admission to a secure psychiatric ward. Therefore, extended history taking, specifically including third-party medical history as well as repeated neurological examination, is paramount and may help to suspect anti-NMDAR encephalitis as the underlying course.
- Third, the diagnostic workup may be unrevealing; for instance, the MRI may be normal in up to two-thirds of cases, and even an inflammatory CSF may be absent [4]. Detection of anti-NMDAR antibodies in CSF appears to be 100 % sensitive, while serum detection yielded a sensitivity of 85 % [4]. Thus, at least anti-NMDAR antibodies in serum should be obtained from patients that are not suitable for LP during the psychotic episode. This is well exemplified in our first patient (RG) in whom the presence of anti-NMDAR serum antibodies led to the diagnosis and initiation of anti-inflammatory treatment.

- Fourth, while the majority of patients is said to recover, anti-inflammatory therapy needs to be initiated and will eventually induce remission. Notably, IVMP may transiently aggravate a psychotic episode, which should not defer from the diagnosis. When first-line immunotherapy (IVMP, IVIg, PE) fails, more aggressive options have to be pursued in nonresponders.

References

1. Jantzen SU, et al. In vitro neuronal network activity in NMDA receptor encephalitis. BMC Neurosci. 2013;14:17.
2. Moscato EH, et al. Acute mechanisms underlying antibody effects in anti-N-methyl-D-aspartate receptor encephalitis. Ann Neurol. 2014;76(1):108–19.
3. Dalmau J, et al. Paraneoplastic anti-N-methyl-D-aspartate receptor encephalitis associated with ovarian teratoma. Ann Neurol. 2007;61(1):25–36.
4. Titulaer MJ, et al. Treatment and prognostic factors for long-term outcome in patients with anti-NMDA receptor encephalitis: an observational cohort study. Lancet Neurol. 2013;12(2):157–65.
5. Kayser MS, et al. Frequency and characteristics of isolated psychiatric episodes in anti–N--methyl-d-aspartate receptor encephalitis. JAMA Neurol. 2013;70(9):1133–9.
6. Gable MS, et al. The frequency of autoimmune N-methyl-D-aspartate receptor encephalitis surpasses that of individual viral etiologies in young individuals enrolled in the California Encephalitis Project. Clin Infect Dis. 2012;54(7):899–904.

Chapter 33
Case Study: Anti-GAD Encephalitis

Helen Walker, Ashwani Jha, Paul Holmes, Thomasin Andrews, Michael Kopelman, and Mervi Pitkanen

The Case

A 58-year-old unemployed white lady was referred to the neuropsychiatry liaison team at a university hospital. She was admitted with confusion, auditory hallucinations, dehydration, malnutrition, upbeating nystagmus and ophthalmoplegia. She had been previously diagnosed with paranoid schizophrenia at the age of 40.

The daughter provided some collateral history regarding her mother's baseline condition prior to recent deterioration and her presentation to accident and emergency. She had been under the care of a community mental health team and had been receiving assistance thrice weekly for her personal care and shopping. She was struggling with climbing stairs and had required lifting assistance. She had occasional

H. Walker, MBChB, MRCPsych (✉)
Department of Neuropsychiatry, St Thomas's Hospital, London, UK
e-mail: Helen.Walker3@slam.nhs.uk; Helen.1.Walker3@kcl.ac.uk

A. Jha, MRCP, PhD
Department of Neurology, St Thomas' Hospital, London, UK
e-mail: ashwani.jha@ucl.ac.uk

P. Holmes, MD, FRCP (UK) • T. Andrews, BSc, MD, FRCP
Department of Neurology, Guy's and St Thomas' NHS Foundation Trust, St Thomas' Hospital, London, UK
e-mail: paul.holmes@gstt.nhs.uk; thomasin.andrews@gstt.nhs.uk

M. Kopelman, PhD, FBPsS, FRCPsych, FMedSci
Department of Academic Neuropsychiatry, King's College London, St Thomas's Hospital, London, UK
e-mail: michael.kopelman@kcl.ac.uk

M. Pitkanen, MBBS, Lic Med, MA, MRC Psych, MD
Department of Neuropsychiatry and Memory Disorders, King's College London, London, UK
e-mail: mervi.pitkanen@kcl.ac.uk

J. Priller, H. Rickards (eds.), *Neuropsychiatry Case Studies*,
DOI 10.1007/978-3-319-42190-2_33

urinary incontinence of unknown cause. Her daughter explained that her mental state had been stable for many years, but 6 weeks prior to admission, she had started to isolate herself, had lost a significant amount of weight, and had left confused voicemails for her. Two weeks before presenting to the hospital, she had refused to see her carers or her daughter. It was the carers who had called an ambulance having found her neglecting her personal care, in a soiled bed, refusing help.

On arrival at the hospital, she was dehydrated with resulting acute kidney injury and hypercalcemia. Regarding her mental state, she was disheveled and guarded and she displayed poor eye contact and psychomotor agitation. She was disorientated in time, place, and person and displayed an incongruous affect with inappropriate smiling.

The patient was rehydrated, and initial investigations found no medical cause for her presentation such as occult infection or pulmonary embolus. She remained disorientated with upbeating nystagmus and a mild restriction of the range of eye movement in all directions (a complex ophthalmoplegia). She reported voices telling her "not to go" to a psychiatric hospital.

Brain imaging including an MRI head was normal. Cerebrospinal fluid analysis was unremarkable, and tests including antibodies to thyroid peroxidase, N-methyl-D-aspartate (NMDA), and voltage-gated potassium channel antibody complex (VGKC) were negative.

Wernicke's encephalopathy, due to a potential history of alcohol misuse or malnutrition, was considered, and intravenous thiamine was given. Risperidone was also commenced at 2 mg once a day and increased after 2 days to 3 mg once a day.

A week later, she was slightly less confused and scored 23/30 on a mini-mental state examination, losing points in the visuospatial and orientation domains. She reported "helpful voices" and a running commentary that she said she had had "for years." Also, there was evidence of confabulation, reporting that she had been in "cafes and restaurants" for the preceding few days. At this point, Wernicke-Korsakoff syndrome was considered a potential working diagnosis.

At 2 weeks into admission, her eye movements improved slightly, although there was some residual nystagmus. Negative symptoms of schizophrenia became evident including abulia, poverty of thought, concrete thinking, and apathy.

A month after admission, she had neurologically deteriorated. The upbeating nystagmus and complex ophthalmoplegia had returned to what it was on admission, and now she had developed a generalized cerebellar syndrome with finger-nose, heel-shin, and gait ataxia. She was more confused – she scored 59/95 on a bedside test of cognitive function (Addenbrooke's Cognitive Examination; some elements were excluded owing to her not having access to her spectacles), and performance in the domains of memory (13/26), fluency (2/14), and visuospatial score (11/16) was particularly poor with relatively preserved attention (16/18) and language (18/21). A neuropsychology assessment revealed a premorbid IQ of 110 with an overall current functioning of 85 (low average), using the WAIS-III, and similarities and matrix reasoning subtests and a borderline visuospatial score (IQ equivalent of 75) using a block design. She also failed a simple executive functioning task (the key search test).

A further course of IV thiamine was given, and the neurology team requested a further paraneoplastic screen including serum antibody testing and a CT scan of the chest, thorax, and abdomen. The auditory hallucinations and negative symptoms of schizophrenia persisted. Risperidone was increased to 4 mg once a day.

She slowly deteriorated during the second month of her admission. An EEG showed "brief bursts of frontal theta activity consistent with an encephalopathy (but of nonspecific etiology). These bursts had no clinical correlate and were not epileptic. Further IV thiamine was given.

Three months into admission, her confusion and eye movements transiently but significantly improved. A repeat test of current full IQ showed an improvement at 100 (using the WAIS-III). However 2 weeks later, she became acutely unwell – she was tachycardic, pyrexial, leukopenic, and hypokalemic. She was given empirical antibiotic treatment, although no source of infection was eventually identified. The medical team stopped the risperidone for 5 days in case it was contributing to her leukopenia. However, she continued to deteriorate, with progressive slowness and poverty of movement interrupted by frequent marked alterations in her mental state. During these episodes, she appeared very distressed and was rolling around in the bed saying that voices were "telling her to die" and were singing to her "we do not care a lot." At other times, she was monosyllabic. Within days she became bedbound, had a startled expression, and developed a mixed movement disorder with both slowness and stiffness of the upper limbs and complex stereotypies involving repeated foot extension. Her nystagmus and ophthalmoplegia worsened. After her bloods had normalized, 0.5 mg risperidone once a day was recommenced and increased gradually to 4 mg once a day, and lorazepam 1 mg once a day was introduced. A serum anti-glutamic acid decarboxylase (GAD) antibody result, which had taken longer than others to process, was very elevated at >50,000 U/ml (normal range 0–5 U/ml).

At 5 months into her admission, her anti-GAD antibodies were repeated and confirmed again a raised titer of >50,000 U/ml – at this point, the working diagnosis became an anti-GAD encephalitis. Intravenous immunoglobulin (IVIg) was begun on the recommendation of the neurology team, but she only tolerated four out of five doses. As she remained very distressed, risperidone was switched to olanzapine 10 mg once a day.

Immediately following the IVIg treatment (which has a delayed onset of action), her condition worsened and she became more distressed, saying she wished to leave. She was detained on the medical ward under Section 2 of the Mental Health Act 1983 (amended in 2007), and olanzapine was increased to 15 mg once a day. At 6 months into her admission, she was dysarthric, and her swallow was impaired requiring a nasogastric tube. However, she was calmer and able to follow simple instructions suggesting a partial response to IVIg treatment and therefore that further immunomodulatory treatment might be successful. The olanzapine was switched to an olanzapine depot, 300 mg fortnightly. She was detained under Section 3 of the Mental Health Act.

Seven months into admission, she underwent further immunomodulation with plasma exchange, although this had to be performed under general anesthetic. At 8 months following admission, she appeared more settled and began to communicate by writing. However she developed a new milder ophthalmoplegia (left eye abduction restriction). Further plasma exchange or IVIg was not administered, and she was transferred to a care home able to provide long-term care for her medical and psychiatric needs.

Regarding personal history, she was the youngest of six children. Her father was reportedly physically and emotionally abusive toward her, her siblings, and her mother. Her father was also allegedly very critical. She was close to her older sister as a child, and she reportedly attempted suicide as a teenager. She was described as an isolated child with few friends. Her mother died at 19 years of age. When she was 17 years old, she was said to have been made to have to leave college to work, and she was a secretary until the age of 30 years.

She was married twice between the ages of 20 and 25 years and 30 and 34 years. Her daughter is from her second marriage. Her second husband was allegedly physically abusive, and there was an injunction order issued against him. Her daughter lived with her until she was 40 years old, which is apparently when her psychotic symptoms began. She then did not have any contact with her daughter for many years.

In terms of psychiatric history, she has had three inpatient admissions to psychiatric wards in 1997, 1999, and 2004. In 1999 she was remanded to prison as she had stolen goods from a shop. She reported at the time that voices were telling her to steal the goods. She was remanded into custody as she failed to attend a magistrates' court hearing. Of note, she was not prescribed medication between 1999 and 2001 and reportedly did not relapse.

Her medical history includes iron-deficiency anemia, and she has no known history of substance misuse. She did not have a history of diabetes.

In summary, a middle-aged white female with a diagnosis of paranoid schizophrenia was an inpatient in a university hospital for approximately 9 months. During this time, she had numerous medical investigations and was subject to neuropsychiatric, neurological, and general medical input. Her neurological complaints (nystagmus, ophthalmoplegia, ataxia, arousal, and movement disorder) fluctuated throughout her admission. Similarly her psychiatric symptoms (auditory persecutory hallucinations, severe anxiety, possible persecutory beliefs) fluctuated and were resistant to antipsychotic treatment. She also experienced global gradual decline in all her higher cognitive functions, and toward the end of her stay, she was largely unable to communicate and required help with all her daily needs. The fluctuations occurred without clear antecedents and may reflect the underlying fluctuating nature of autoimmune disease. There was partial evidence of a transient benefit from neuromodulatory treatments, but she was discharged with significant residual functional impairment.

What Did I Learn from This Case?

This case highlights some of the key dilemmas in psychiatric and neurological practice that have come about following recent advances in autoimmune encephalopathies.

The patient's initial presentation was quite dramatic with marked neglect, malnutrition, and dehydration in addition to her psychiatric features. In this context, the discovery of upbeating nystagmus and initial anterograde memory loss with confabulation made Wernicke-Korsakoff syndrome the most likely diagnosis. However, she only partially responded to IV thiamine, and she received repeated courses throughout her admission. However, unusually for Wernicke-Korsakoff syndrome, after treatment for about a month into her admission, her neurological syndrome progressed with the development of additional cerebellar features (limb and gait ataxia). The diagnosis of Wernicke-Korsakoff was challenged, and this prompted the search for paraneoplastic and other autoimmune causes of a cerebellar syndrome, but unfortunately her anti-GAD antibody results were not available until a few months later. Three months into her admission, she temporarily improved for a couple of weeks but then dramatically worsened with new features that were again inconsistent with pure Wernicke-Korsakoff syndrome. She developed an unexplained pyrexia, a markedly fluctuating mental state, a startled expression, and eventually a mixed movement disorder with stereotypies. These features strongly favored an autoimmune encephalopathy, and this was confirmed when anti-GAD antibodies were detected in her serum.

Over the last 15 years, the characterization of autoimmune encephalopathies has markedly matured mainly due to the discovery of antibodies in the serum and CSF of patients with acute encephalopathies [1]. These patients can present with psychiatric features initially before going on to develop red flag symptoms such as pyrexia, seizures, and movement disorders. Additionally if diagnosis is delayed, treatment is likely to be less effective.

The commonest antibodies present in the sera of such patients are N-methyl-D-aspartate (NMDA) and voltage-gated potassium channel antibody complex [1]: both are thought to be pathogenic because they are cell surface antigens in the central nervous system, and in some cases serum levels correlate with disease severity [1]. In our case, these antibodies and many others tested were negative, but anti-GAD antibodies were very high. However, whether anti-GAD antibodies cause autoimmune encephalopathy is debated and is now explored further.

Glutamic acid decarboxylase (GAD) is a presynaptic enzyme responsible for the synthesis of GABA in the central nervous system. In 1988, Solimena et al. discovered antibodies to GAD in a patient with type 1 diabetes and stiff-person syndrome (a progressive autoimmune neurological condition causing characteristic muscle stiffness due to abnormal continuous muscle activity) [2]. Since then, antibodies to the smaller 65 kDa isoform of GAD (called GAD65) have been shown to be present at low levels in patients with type 1 diabetes only and at high levels in those with stiff-person syndrome only [3]. In 2008 Saiz et al. showed that anti-GAD antibodies were also present in the serum and CSF of some patients with subacute limbic encephalitis and cerebellar syndrome as well as some with chronic epilepsy of up to 34-year duration, leading to speculation that these antibodies could potentially be responsible for varied acute and chronic neurological syndromes [4]. However, unlike NMDA and VGKC complex, GAD is an intracellular antigen. This is important because it has led some to speculate that the antibody may be a bystander rather than pathogenic [5]. In any case, it remains a useful marker for autoimmune CNS disease.

Data on treatment is sparse and limited to anti-GAD-positive stiff-person syndrome; the best evidence is for immunomodulation with intravenous immunoglobulin [6], although this study had only 16 participants. Corticosteroids, plasma exchange, and azathioprine have all been anecdotally successful. Rituximab is a monoclonal antibody against B cells and has gained recent favor in other autoimmune encephalopathies and also been anecdotally successful in stiff-person syndrome [1, 7]. Our patient partially responded to these treatments, but they were given quite late on in the course of her symptoms.

Finally, it is important to note that while anti-GAD encephalitis explains most of her later features she may well have had an additional thiamine deficiency at the start of her hospital admission. What is more intriguing is whether a low-grade anti-GAD syndrome could have caused her previous psychiatric symptoms particularly as she seemed to have had unexplained past episodes of deterioration and uncharacteristic behavior. However, this must remain as speculation.

References

1. Vincent A, Bien CG, Irani SR, Waters P. Autoantibodies associated with diseases of the CNS: new developments and future challenges. Lancet Neurol. 2011;10(8):759–72.
2. Solimena M, Folli F, Denis-Donini S, Comi GC, Pozza G, De Camilli P, Vicari AM. Autoantibodies to glutamic acid decarboxylase in a patient with stiff-man syndrome, epilepsy, and type I diabetes mellitus. N Engl J Med. 1988;318(16):1012–20.
3. Hadavi S, Noyce A, Leslie R, Giovannoni G. Stiff person syndrome. Pract Neurol. 2011;11: 272–82.
4. Saiz A, Blanco Y, Sabater L, González F, Bataller L, Casamitjana R, Ramió-Torrentà L, Graus F. Spectrum of neurological syndromes associated with glutamic acid decarboxylase antibodies: diagnostic clues for this association. Brain. 2008;131(10):2553–63.
5. Vincent A. Stiff, twitchy or wobbly: are GAD antibodies pathogenic? Brain. 2008;131(Pt 10):2536–7.
6. Dalakas MC, Fujii M, Li M, Lutfi B, Kyhos J, McElroy B. High-dose intravenous immune globulin for stiff-person syndrome. N Engl J Med. 2001;345(26):1870–6.
7. McKeon A, Robinson MT, McEvoy KM, Matsumoto JY, Lennon VA, Ahlskog JE, Pittock SJ. Stiff-man syndrome and variants: clinical course, treatments, and outcomes. Arch Neurol. 2012;69(2):230–8.

Other Sources Consulted

Hodges J. Addenbrooke's Cognitive Examination – ACE-R final revised version A. 2005.
Wechsler D. Wechsler Adult Intelligence Scale® – Third Edition\(WAIS®-III), 1997.

Part VI
Organic Psychosis and Organic Personality Disorders

Chapter 34
Animals in My Tummy

Fernando Lázaro Perlado

J.M.C. is a 49-year-old right-handed unemployed man who was admitted to our unit as he could no longer be cared for at home since his psychotic illness had worsened. He presented with kinesthetic hallucinations (felt animals in his stomach) and claimed that his words were escaping through his mouth. He described "pain" in his lips and around his mouth. In order to prevent his "words from escaping," he would hold a spoon in his mouth and would continuously look at a book as if he were reading, however always looking at the same page. There were some episodes where he could not find his way back home, not being able of giving an account of his whereabouts afterwards, and at one point, he was given a GPS locator so he could be found. He was very distressed and was unable to complete his basic ADLs without supervision and support. He presented with no focal neurological signs.

Background History

He was born at home from a normal delivery and, on his account, achieved normal developmental milestones. He told us that he had no memories from his childhood, stating that he did not go to school for very long, attending some kind of "academy." He said that he only worked for 3 months, spending most of his time "sleeping" at home. He lived with his elderly parents and a younger sister, who suffers from depression. He has two other sisters (one of whom suffers from anxiety) and a brother. We were told that his difficulties started when he was 21 years old and had to leave home to complete his military service which was mandatory at the time.

F. Lázaro Perlado, LMS, MSc, MRCPsych
Department of Neuropsychiatry, R.S.M.B. Hospital de Bermeo,
Bermeo, Bizkaia, Spain

Clínica Indautxu, C/ Gordóniz 9, 48010 Bilbao, Bizkaia, Spain
e-mail: fernando.lazaroperlado@osakidetza.eus; drflazaro@movistar.es

J. Priller, H. Rickards (eds.), *Neuropsychiatry Case Studies*,
DOI 10.1007/978-3-319-42190-2_34

The following year, in 1988, he was diagnosed with paranoid schizophrenia. Since then, he has had many admissions to the psychiatric unit. Different treatments were tried over the years with virtually no success. He developed hepatotoxicity with clozapine, having the drug to be withdrawn, presented with prolonged confusional states after ECT, and also showed a "paradoxical reaction" to haloperidol with worsening of his clinical presentation, whenever the drug was administered. In time, he slowly lost functional ability and autonomy, becoming dependent upon his supportive family.

Examination

Mental state examination revealed a young Caucasian man, casually dressed however somewhat disheveled. He maintained fleeting eye contact and showed psychomotor retardation. He spoke in a low and monotonous voice about his problems, not being able to redirect his interest to other matters. He came across as euthymic with a flat affect. He denied suicidal ideation intention or planning. He referred having animals in his stomach, he could feel them moving in it, and later identified them as a cat and a dog. He also reported that words were escaping through his mouth. There were no auditory hallucinations. He showed no insight into his predicament.

He was treated with an atypical antipsychotic, which he could also have as if needed (p.r.n.). It was noticed that whenever he became distressed and focused in his delusions and hallucinations and was given the p.r.n. antipsychotic, he would become even more distressed. However, if oral lorazepam was administered, it would have a clear calming effect.

Investigations

1. Scalp EEG (21.08.2012): Reported as normal.
2. Scalp EEG (29.08.2012): Detected two episodes, lasting 35–40 s, compatible with left posterior temporal ictal events. Interictal electric pattern within normal range.
3. Epilepsy Unit video EEG monitoring (07.01.2013): Detects rapid rhythm secondary to medication. They describe multiple episodes compatible with non-epileptic paroxistic events.
4. Brain MRI (19.10.2012): Multiple cerebral cavernomas were detected. The biggest one measured 1.5 cm in length and was located in the left temporo-occipital junction (see Figs. 34.1 and 34.2), with another sizeable one (0.6×0.98 cm) located in the right cerebellar hemisphere (Fig. 34.3). Other smaller cavernomas were detected in the left anterior cingulate cortex, right medial frontal lobe, and right posterior cortex. The mesial temporal regions seem to be unaffected. No other abnormalities are detected.

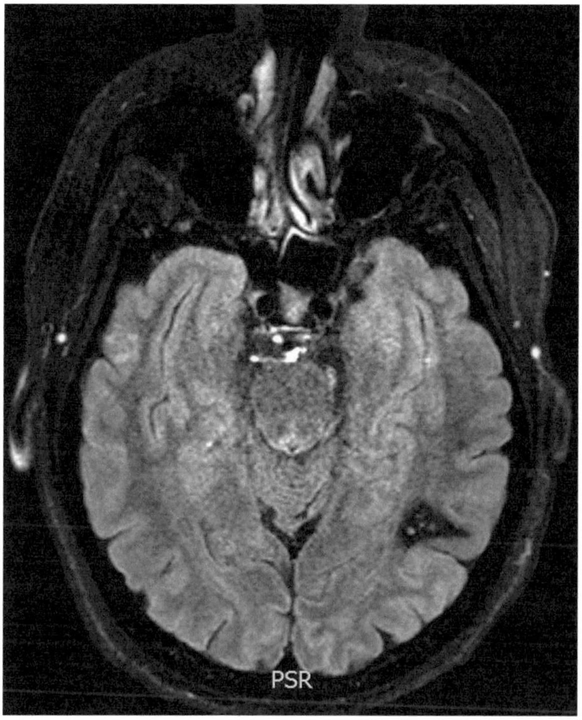

Fig. 34.1 Axial cranial MRI, FLAIR sequence, detecting a 1.5 cm long cavernoma in the left temporal-parietal-occipital junction

Progress in the Ward

Initially, the patient presented episodes of agitation with psychotic symptoms, which did not respond to antipsychotic medication and worsened if its frequency of administration (p.r.n. dosage) was increased. He was started on levetiracetam but showed behavioral problems (including physical aggression when not allowed to smoke during his admission in the Epilepsy Unit), which disappeared when changed into carbamazepine plus clobazam.

He was assessed by the neurologists, who were of the opinion that it was very unlikely that his clinical presentation was of ictal etiology; thus, they recommended to withdraw the antiepileptic drugs (AED) and to continue assessing the course of his cavernomatosis.

Complete withdrawal of the AED could not be achieved due to clear worsening of the clinical picture (increased agitation and distress, interrupted pattern of sleep, and continuous references to words escaping through his mouth and animals in his stomach). Hence, we proceeded to reinstate the AED plus antipsychotic medication that would not lower the seizure threshold (quetiapine and amisulpride).

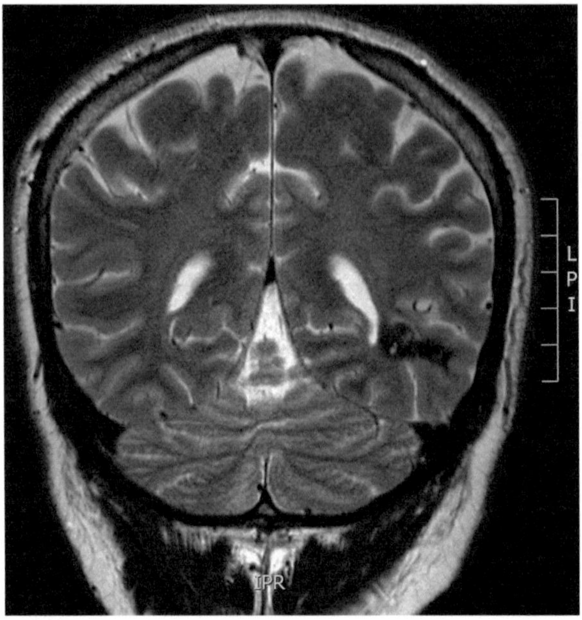

Fig. 34.2 Coronal cranial MRI, T2 sequence, showing the same cavernoma

The patient improved dramatically and was able to start spending time at home, which was gradually increased to a 4-day-a-week "on leave" period plus summer holidays.

We agreed with his family that he would be discharged home with home support an hour a day and daily attendance to a day hospital, where he would receive psychiatric follow-up and his medication would be organized (dossette box) and monitored.

Summary

We have presented the case of a man who, for over 20 years, had been diagnosed with paranoid schizophrenia and treated accordingly, sometimes with some extraordinary therapeutic measures (ECT, clozapine). Despite all these efforts, his clinical presentation barely changed; he could not function independently and was admitted on multiple occasions.

The fact that he presented with "paradoxical reactions" to antipsychotic drugs should have been taken into account earlier, since we believe that overlooking this sign delayed making the correct diagnosis and starting adequate treatment.

The first scalp EEG (performed before the MRI) showed what is described as left posterior temporal ictal events although of short duration. This was not detected

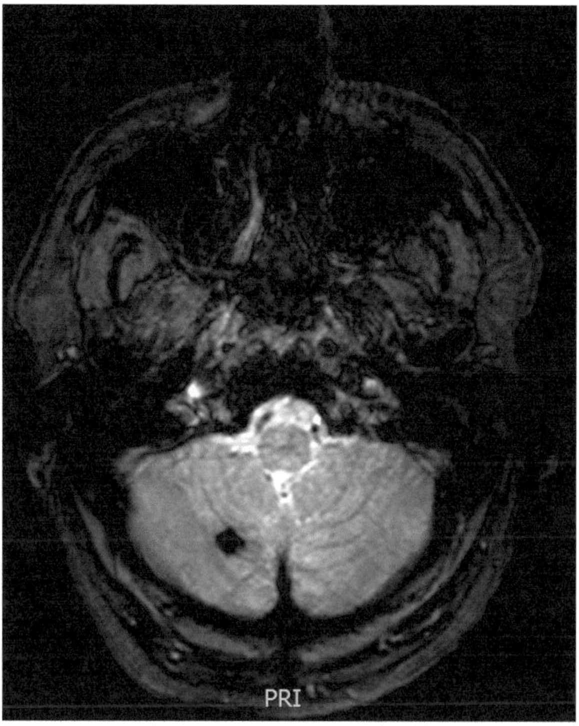

Fig. 34.3 Axial cranial MRI, T2 fat-saturated sequence, showing a smaller cavernoma (0.66×0.98 cm) in the right cerebellar lobule

again in further EEGs and its clinical relevance was even questioned later on. However, structural neuroimaging detected the presence of multiple cavernomas in his brain. We believe that the fact that the largest one is situated in the same area where an EEG detected abnormal electrical activity is relevant to the presentation of this case and its course.

Differential Diagnosis

1. Paranoid schizophrenia

   Although he fulfilled some of the diagnostic criteria for paranoid schizophrenia (delusions, hallucinations, deteriorated social and personal functioning, etc.), it had to be obviously discarded in the presence of the neuroimaging and EEG findings.
2. Ictal psychosis

   The initial working diagnosis was that of an "organic psychosis" of probable epileptic etiology, of temporal lobe origin [1]. We felt that his feeling of having animals in his stomach was compatible with his own personal interpretation of the feelings associated with an epileptic aura (epigastric or visceral), which was accompanied with fear and distress because his words are escaping through his mouth. As we got to know the patient and his symptoms and signs better, we felt that his ideas of the words escaping through his mouth could well be his way of interpreting paresthetic and perhaps painful sensations, congruent with a parietal focus [2], which complicated matters even further.

3. Organic psychosis secondary to familial multiple cavernomatosis
   Based on his clinical presentation, neurological assessment, neuroimaging, and EEG findings, our final diagnosis was that of an organic psychosis secondary to familial multiple cavernomatosis. Although we acknowledge that a diagnosis of epilepsy (or ictal psychosis) would be difficult to support, the successful treatment encompassed not only antipsychotic medication but also AED in order to modulate the neuronal electrical activity, which very likely is altered by the presence of the cavernomas.

Learning Points

- Careful evaluation and assessment of every patient is of paramount importance.
- All symptoms and signs have to be taken into account, and one must make an effort to understand their possible causes in order to make the correct diagnosis and treat accordingly.
- If a patient does not respond to treatment (using current guidelines and protocols), the differential diagnosis has to be reconsidered and appropriate investigations ordered.

References

1. Temporal lobe epilepsies, in chapter 12: the symptomatic and probably symptomatic focal epilepsies. In: Panayiotopoulos CP, editor. The epilepsies: seizures, syndromes and management. Chipping Norton: Bladon Medical Publishing; 2005. p. 362–93.
2. Parietal lobe epilepsies, in chapter 12: the symptomatic and probably symptomatic focal epilepsies. In: Panayiotopoulos CP, editor. The epilepsies: seizures, syndromes and management. Chipping Norton: Bladon Medical Publishing; 2005. p. 410–16.

Chapter 35
Personality Changes After Encephalitis: When "Organic Personality Disorder" Is Not Enough

Maria del Mar Amador and Thomas Mauras

F.C. is a previously healthy 21-year-old female presenting a challenging emotional and behavioral disorder starting at the age of 19. At that age, while attending university, she started complaining of concentration difficulties. Subsequent ophthalmoplegia with bilateral ptosis, abnormal jaw movements, and difficulties in swallowing prompted neurological evaluation. Brain magnetic resonance imaging (MRI) revealed large bilateral lesions in deep brain structures (Fig. 35.1). Cell count in cerebrospinal fluid (CSF) was 16 lymphocytes. One single CSF sample was positive for anti-GAD testing (Oxford Laboratory), but following tests remained negative for this or other antibodies, as well as an extensive inflammatory, infectious, and neoplastic workup. Autoimmune encephalitis was suspected. Initial treatment was administered in the intensive care unit because of altered level of consciousness. It involved high-dose corticoid therapy, plasma exchanges, and intravenous immune globulins. Clinical evolution was satisfactory with rapid improvement of neurological symptoms. The first behavioral changes occurred during the intensive care unit (ICU) stay in the form of stereotypic handwashing without intrusive thoughts, hyperphagia, and akathisia. Three weeks after admission, she was transferred to a neurological ward and discharged after 2 further weeks.

M. del Mar Amador, MD (✉)
Département de Neurologie, Groupe Hospitalier Pitié-Salpêtrière, Paris, France
e-mail: mariadelmar.amador@psl.aphp.fr

T. Mauras, MD
Service de Psychiatrie, Institut Hospitalo-Universitaire de l'Institut du Cerveau et de la Moelle Epinière, Groupe Hospitalier Pitié-Salpêtrière, Paris, France
e-mail: thomas.mauras@psl.aphp.fr

J. Priller, H. Rickards (eds.), *Neuropsychiatry Case Studies*,
DOI 10.1007/978-3-319-42190-2_35

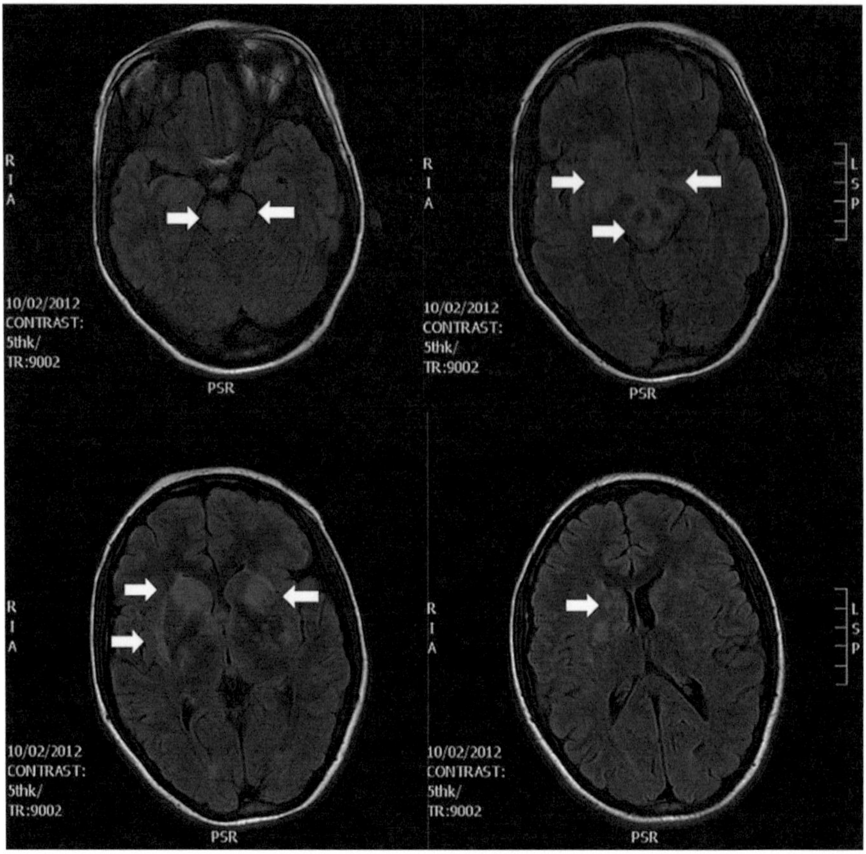

Fig. 35.1 Axial T2 fluid-attenuated inversion recovery (FLAIR)-weighted images of brain MRI in the acute encephalitic phase. Hyperintense T2 lesions are present in both caudate nucleus and lenticular nucleus, both hypothalamus and internal temporal region, as well as both cerebral peduncles (see *white arrows*). Gadolinium enhancement was seen on striatum, anterior commissure, and right temporal intern region

Background History

According to F.C., she was an unremarkable teen. She was a good student at high school and graduated in time. She started studying history at the university. She lived with her parents, who both worked at a hospital. She had an 11-year-old younger brother. She emphasized the fact that her life before the illness was uneventfull without pitfalls. After the onset of the neurological illness, F.C. recently began music courses but reported irregular attendance. At present time she had been for the last 4 months in an intense relationship with a 40-year-old man. In the last year, she frequently engaged in romantic relationships that never lasted more than 5 months. She reported that in spite of developing affectionate relationships with these men, she was not able to remain faithful.

Progress

In the months following discharge, unusual sexual disinhibition and risk-seeking behavior were reported. According to her, she could not avoid bringing about situations in order to have sexual intercourses with unknown males, a behavior which occurred frequently (every other day). Growing anxiety led to panic attacks several times daily. Convulsions developed and after epilepsy workup, the diagnosis of a non-epileptic attack disorder was made. The patient reported afterwards that she triggered the "attacks" to gain the attention of potential sexual partners. The patient was eventually raped.

Six months after discharge from the neurological ward, the patient attempted for the first time to commit suicide by defenestration. Compulsions and impulsive behavior were noted. A course of paroxetine (20 mg daily) was tried for 3 months without any change in mood or behavior. Aripiprazole (5 mg daily) and sodium valproate (1,000 mg daily) were then added in the psychiatry department. The patient was referred to the neurology clinic, and a further series of plasma exchanges was performed, with temporary improvement of behavioral symptoms.

During the following 18 months, the patient was repeatedly hospitalized, twice in a closed ward, because of seven further suicide attempts. In all cases, suicide attempts were performed in the presence of witnesses who retained her from defenestration or from jumping onto subway rails. She afterwards criticized her own acts, confirmed the absence of a wish to die, and qualified her actions as an "appeal for help." Antidepressants were introduced and a psychiatric and psychological follow-up began. In psychiatric interviews, she described her father as a distant person. Her relationship with him was difficult since he spent most of the time at work, and she reported suffering from the feeling of valorousness and unworthiness to her father. She subsequently asserted feeling the need to have sex in order to test her attractiveness and ultimately bolster her value.

Further neurological evaluation disclosed no inflammatory activity, so that no other immunomodulatory treatment was administered. She was hospitalized for a routine follow-up examination in our neuropsychiatric ward.

Examination

F.C. was well groomed. She was alert and cooperative. Contact was superficial and disinhibited. She was self-centered, constantly sought attention, and acted overly seductive and dramatic. She showed quickly changing emotions, low tolerance of frustration, and altogether emotional immaturity. The patient spoke about her situation and particularly about sexual aspects and the experience of rape in detail. Her thought process was normal. Thought content was diminished (sexual content). No psychotic symptoms or delusions were present. Insight was full. Judgment was fair. Ability to concentrate was diminished. Mood was slightly depressed. She described suffering from a chronic feeling of emptiness. A noticeable anxiety corresponded to obsessions and was expressed through frequent and overly theatrical "panic attacks." The initially reported hyperphagia had resolved, and her eating behavior was normal. Night sleep was good. She complained of fatigue almost every day, leading to the restriction of her activities. Sexual drive was nevertheless enhanced. She stated having the need to please, to feel physical and most of all mental attraction. According to her, she acted that way in order to feel love and to exist. She felt guilty about that. There was some degree of motor restlessness.

Her neurological physical exam revealed tremor of the upper extremities and head, ataxic gait, and mild dysarthria.

Further Investigations

Neuropsychological evaluation was performed (Table 35.1). Main abnormalities involved behavioral aspects including impulsivity, lack of inhibition, and sexual conduct. Concentration and selective attention were the only cognitive functions found to be deficient. A follow-up brain MRI showed persistent T2-hyperintense lesions in deep brain structures (Fig. 35.2). Single-photon emission computed tomography (SPECT) was normal. Electrophysiological recording of tremor disclosed a mixed origin (brain stem postural and rest tremor with a psychogenic component).

Table 35.1 Neuropsychological assessment

Areas	Tests	Results
Attention	Hayling sentence completion test, d2 test of attention	Deficit in maintaining attention
Executive functions	Stroop test, mental flexibility at trail making test (A and B), modified wisconsin card sorting test, phonetic and semantic verbal fluency	Preserved, particularly inhibition, good rules adherence and deduction skills
Memory	Free and cued selective reminding rest with immediate recall	Visual and verbal memory were intact
Instrumental functions, language	Testing for constructive apraxia, rey figure copy, DO80-picture-naming test, and orthography test	Normal
Social cognition	Mini-social cognition and emotional assessment	Facial emotions were well recognized although sadness was often mistaken with a neutral face
Impulsivity	Barratt impulsiveness scale-11, plutchick scale	Scales showed a trend towards an increased impulsivity
Apathy	Stakstein apathy scale (filled out by relatives)	Modestly positive

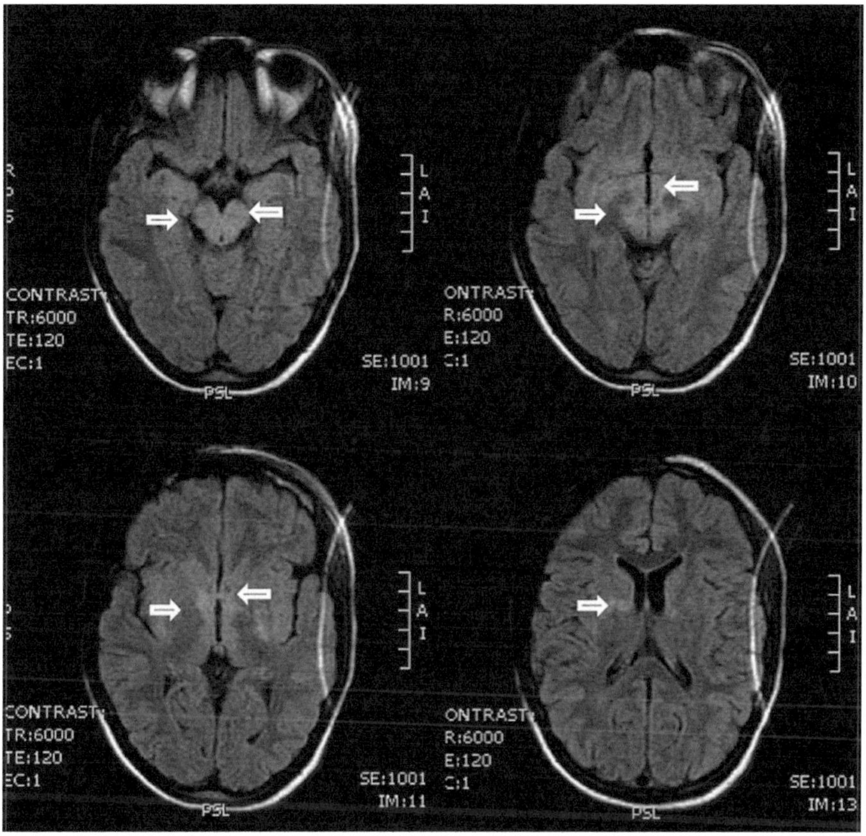

Fig. 35.2 Axial T2 FLAIR-weighted images 2 years after initial MRI showing persistent hyperintense lesions in the mesencephalic region, surrounding the third ventricle and the aqueduct of Sylvius as well as in the basal ganglia. No gadolinium enhancement was found

Diagnosis

F.C. had a complex presentation with disinhibition and risk-taking behavior, instability of the self, and preoccupation with real or imagined abandonment, associated with impairments in interpersonal functioning. These impairments were relatively stable over time and consistent across situations and had a significant impact on daily life. All of these symptoms met the criteria for borderline personality disorder [1]. Consistent with the diagnosis of organic personality disorder, the symptoms were unmasked and intrusive only after the encephalitis. On the one hand, the severity of the neurological illness and the extent of the brain lesions, probably disrupting the limbic circuitry, plead for an organic origin of the disabling behavior. On the other hand, her capacity of insight leading to reassessment of her formerly idealized childhood points to a previously slightly borderline functioning. Notably, in spite of the extent of the brain lesions and contrasting with the severity of the behavioral abnormalities, no cognitive function was affected except attention. In particular, cognitive impulsivity was preserved in neuropsychological testing.

Differential Diagnosis

Klüver-Bucy syndrome is a classical neuropsychiatric phenotype. It occurs after diverse types of brain damage affecting both amygdalae and their cortical connections. Encephalitis, particularly herpetic, is a well-recognized cause of this syndrome. Our patient presented a probable dysimmune encephalitis. Her risk behaviors could be interpreted as a defective fear-adaptive behavior. She also presented an abnormal sexual behavior and some degree of attention deficit. However, many features of Klüver-Bucy syndrome were absent (Table 35.2). Her hypersexuality was not indiscriminate since she reported choosing men she considered attractive. Furthermore, there were no visible lesions in the medial temporal lobes and no stigmata of amygdala dysfunction in neuropsychological testing [2].

What Did I Learn from This Case?

One interesting point is that neuroanatomical correlations to symptoms, routinely used in neurology, may also apply to some psychiatric symptoms, as revealed by the obsessive-compulsive disorder of our patient in the ICU. Obsessive-compulsive symptoms have been related to other neurological pathologies disrupting the basal ganglia circuitry [3].

This case is a good example of the dynamic process underlying the construction and maintenance of personality. F.C. is a young woman whose personality was not fixed by the time of the neurological illness. The encephalitis was a double aggression in this context. First, damaging key structures such as the basal ganglia implicated in emotional and behavioral regulation. Second, this health event was

Table 35.2 Main Klüver-Bucy syndrome features as compared with patient's features

Klüver-Bucy syndrome features	Features presented by the patient
Hyperorality with hyperphagia	Only in the acute phase
Memory deficits	None
Visual agnosia	None
Aphasia	None
Distractibility	Deficit in maintaining attention
Hypersexuality	Hypersexuality (but not indiscriminate)
Defective fear-adaptive behavior	Risk-taking behavior (but no difficulties in facial recognition of fear)

undeniably a psychological trauma leading to a narcissistic wound. She considered herself as a miracle girl and this radically changed the direction of her life values. Her sexual impulsivity might be regarded as a strategy of coping, as it has been proposed in the borderline personality disorder [4].

In this complex context, it is difficult to sort out what belongs to each component. Incline towards an exclusive lesional cause of the symptoms implies accepting that this particular brain damage pattern perfectly mimics borderline personality disorder. Even further, this could be interpreted as the proof of the concept that borderline personality is underlined by specific reorganizations of brain circuits [5].

References

1. Gunderson JG. Borderline personality disorder. N Engl J Med. 2014;364(21):2037–42.
2. Hayman LA, Rexer JL, Pavol MA, Strite D, Meyers CA. Klüver-Bucy syndrome after bilateral selective damage of amygdala and its cortical connections. J Neuropsychiatry Clin Neurosci. 1998;10:354–8.
3. Walterfang M, Yucel M, Walker R, Evans A, Bader B, Ng A, et al. Adolescent obsessive compulsive disorder heralding chorea-acanthocytosis. Mov Disord. 2008;23(3):422–5.
4. Sansone RA, Sansone LA. Sexual behavior in borderline personality. Innov Clin Neurosci. 2011;8(2):14–8.
5. Krause-Utz A, Winter D, Niedtfeld I, Schmahl C. The latest neuroimaging findings in borderline personality disorder. Curr Psychiatry Rep. 2014;16(3):438.

Chapter 36
Case Vignette. Brain Injury Can Make One Better!

Kanu Achinivu

SS is a 58-year-old woman who had a history of anxiety and depression and severe gambling addiction. At the age of 54, she was hit by a car at a zebra crossing while walking to local shops and as a result suffered a severe traumatic brain injury. Her Glasgow Coma Scale (GCS) was very depressed at 6/15, and she had a protracted period of posttraumatic amnesia (PTA) of greater than 2 weeks. A CT scan showed bilateral small acute subdural hematomas and multiple contusions especially in both temporal lobes as well as fractures of the skull vault and base of the skull. She was treated conservatively in the hospital and discharged to a local rehabilitation unit where she demonstrated significant cognitive, emotional, and neurobehavioral problems. She refused interventions and was deemed to lack insight. She made gradual improvement though showed a lack of insight into her difficulties and lacked awareness of her neuropsychiatric problems and functional ability. She was discharged home and subsequently refused further carer or rehabilitation input.

When seen in clinic, SS denied experiencing any major problems with looking after herself. She also denied any difficulties with cooking or shopping. She admitted that at times, she could be forgetful though did not seem unduly worried about this. At the time, she was living with a boyfriend who she had met after her brain injury and she described a good relationship.

Collateral history provided by a family member indicated that SS had not gambled since the accident though she had had a go at the machines but "could not figure them out." She had however, since the accident, come home with various men, something she had not done before. She had also shown inappropriate affection to a male carer, which led to the agency sending only female carers. However, these behaviors had somewhat improved over the years since the accident especially

K. Achinivu, MBBS, MSc, MRCPsych
Department of Neuropsychiatry, National Centre for Mental Health, The Barberry, Birmingham, UK
e-mail: kanu.achinivu@bsmhft.nhs.uk

J. Priller, H. Rickards (eds.), *Neuropsychiatry Case Studies*,
DOI 10.1007/978-3-319-42190-2_36

after she met her current partner. Her family member felt that she lacked motivation and drive though this was becoming better.

A phone call to her partner described her as someone who was "very distant" and experiencing mood swings regularly. She was said to be "very nasty" and then "alright" and could become aggressive "if you speak to her the wrong way." He also highlighted that she suffered from significant lack of motivation and would "sit staring out of the window" if not prompted. He stated that her short-term memory was poor and she also had significant problems with long-term memory. He did not consider her to be depressed or anxious.

Background History

SS was employed and enjoyed a relatively stable married life until she was made redundant. She soon developed a depressive disorder and started to gamble. Her gambling progressively got out of hand as she was repeatedly in debt of large sums of money and got into disagreements with family members and her husband. Her family members had to intervene to pay off her excessive debts. She required care from local psychiatric services and received a variety of interventions for her mental health difficulties including various psychological interventions and psychiatric treatments like antidepressants, anxiolytic drugs, hypnotic drugs, and low-dose antipsychotic drugs. She also enrolled in Gamblers Anonymous. She required a lot of input from primary care services as well as secondary care mental health services due to her problems. Her marriage eventually broke down due to her gambling problems and excessive debts.

There was no family history of epilepsy, psychiatric disorder, or degenerative disorder.

Examination

Mental state examination revealed a middle-aged woman who appeared older than her age. She appeared slightly unkempt and fatigued. She was subdued in mood and seemed rather unconcerned about her memory difficulties. Her answers to questions were short with many questions answered with "I don't know." She was alert, though not oriented to time. Her memory for events before the accident seemed somewhat impaired, and she seemed to have difficulty recalling events that had happened since the accident. It was noted that while she provided some answers, which seemed logical, many of these were found to be wrong. Neurological examination revealed loss of sense of smell.

Investigations

A neuropsychology assessment was requested. Routine MRI showed changes compatible with her TBI.

Progress

Neuropsychology evaluation demonstrated significant acquired cognitive impairments in all areas of cognitive functioning including intellectual functioning, memory, attention and concentration, and executive functioning, with memory and working memory being particularly affected. It was also felt that SS demonstrated a complete lack of insight into the extent of her difficulties. It was felt that she would struggle to live independently and a rehabilitation program should be instituted.

It was also felt that there might be a degree of confabulation. The family views were that SS seemed to be much better since the accident as she stopped gambling and as she was not as disabled by depression and anxiety as before.

SS and her partner did not think that any rehabilitation was necessary and felt that they were managing generally well together. In particular, SS was not keen to engage with any intervention.

Diagnosis

A diagnosis of an organic personality change/disorder following brain injury was made according to the ICD-10 diagnostic criteria. A diagnosis of a specific memory disorder was also considered due to impaired recent and remote memory as well as confabulation.

What Did I Learn from This Case?

Personality disorders are generally understood to cause significant problems to society in general, and most doctors will be familiar with the Phineas Gage case in which a brain injury led to severe impulsivity and aggression. However, this case shows that though a diagnosis of an organic personality change/disorder was made due to the significant changes from premorbid behavior, it does suggest that her personality change seemed to have been of some benefit.

Most professionals involved in SS's case were of the opinion that she seemed to function better overall following her brain injury compared to pre-accident. She had stopped gambling, seemed to have settled into some form of routine with her new partner, and experienced less depression and anxiety. As a result, her dependence on the health service had markedly reduced, and it was felt that her overall level of disability was lower compared to pre-accident. She did, however, have significant cognitive impairments as a result of the brain injury.

Behavioral impairments following a brain injury can present as an increase, a decrease, or a dysregulation of behavior. This case showed a decrease in goal-directed behavior, which can occur on a continuum of severity ranging from mildly diminished motivation to akinetic mutism in severe cases. While behavioral problems following brain injury can be an obstacle to engaging in rehabilitation and need to be identified and treated, in some cases, the behavioral change can be of benefit, taking into account the premorbid personality of the particular patient.

Bibliography

1. Harlow JM. Recovery from the passage of an iron bar through the head. Publ Mass Med Soc. 1868;2:327–46.
2. Greve KW, Sherwin E, Stanford MS, et al. Personality and neurocognitive correlates of impulsive aggression in long-term survivors of severe traumatic brain injury. Brain Inj. 2001;15: 255–62.
3. Daffner KR, Mesulam MM, Holcomb PJ, et al. Disruption of attention to novel events after frontal lobe injury in humans. J Neurol Neurosurg Psychiatry. 2000;68:18–24.
4. Kalivas PW, Volkaw ND. The neural basis of addiction: a pathology of motivation and choice. Am J Psychiatry. 2005;162:1403–13.

Part VII
Other Neuropsychiatric Disorders

Chapter 37
Psychosis Following Traumatic Brain Injury

Tarek Zghoul and Kieran O'Driscoll

A Caucasian female, currently in her 30s, sustained a traumatic brain injury (TBI) secondary to a road traffic accident. She had no memories of the events. The severe TBI caused frontal lobe and cerebellar contusions, a subarachnoid hemorrhage, and diffuse axonal injury (DAI). She was found unconscious with a Glasgow Coma Scale of 3/15 and suffered from post-traumatic amnesia greater than two weeks. She underwent several surgical procedures including eye surgery. As a result of these injuries, she was rendered physically and mentally impaired with immediate detrimental effects on her daily activities of living.

In the months and years following the accident, complex neurobehavioral deficits began to emerge. Three years following the TBI, she became socially isolated, erratic, intolerant, displaying enhanced verbal aggression, agitation, and impulsivity as well as ill-judged behavior lacking insight. She abused alcohol. Neuropsychologically, she demonstrated very significant cognitive issues including short-term memory impairment and marked executive function deficits. She displayed non-epileptic seizures, having had no previous history of fits. Her presentation became more complex with the appearance of psychotic features. She began expressing the firm and unshakable belief that she had a microchip implanted in her brain and that this was controlling her. She remained convinced of the presence of this electronic device even after having been shown the results of neuroimaging

T. Zghoul, MBChB, PhD (✉)
Department of Psychiatry, Oxford University, Warneford Hospital, Oxford, UK
e-mail: tarek.zghoul@psych.ox.ac.uk

K. O'Driscoll, FRCPsych
David Lewis Centre, Cheshire, UK
e-mail: kieranjudeodriscoll@yahoo.co.uk

J. Priller, H. Rickards (eds.), *Neuropsychiatry Case Studies*,
DOI 10.1007/978-3-319-42190-2_37

studies, further insisting that she wanted the chip surgically removed. She believed she was a victim of ongoing illegal experiments carried out under the auspices of a global organization. She stated that her eyes had been operated on illegally and that this was a breach of her human rights. Furthermore, she expressed the belief that she was being followed by people belonging to a certain national group and that they were trying to shoot her. She had no insight into her mental illness, denying that she had a mental health problem, stating that she was being forcibly injected with medication without medical justification. She believed that she was fit to return to her pre-TBI way of living with no insight into her severe mental and physical disability.

Background

She had a normal birth and development, reaching all her milestones on time. She had no reported issues at home, school, college, her social circle, or relationships. She eventually worked in the service industry and excelled professionally. Prior to the TBI, she had no past psychiatric or medical history. There was no family history of mental illness. Premorbidly, she was described as confident, popular, and the "life and soul of the party."

Examination

In addition to paranoid delusions, she believed that she was being persecuted by a certain group of people wanting to shoot her. She firmly held a belief that she had a microchip implanted in her brain, exerting control over her. These thoughts emerged 3–4 years following the TBI. She complained of symptoms of depression. Changes to her behavior were evident. She became socially isolated, displayed increased aggression, and showed reduced lack of impulse control. Further, her cognitive and executive function demonstrated severe deficits with impaired short-term memory, inability to recall new information, impaired problem-solving skills, and mental inflexibility with a rigid and preservative thinking pattern. She had no insight into her mental health condition.

Investigation

Neuroimaging demonstrated bilateral occipital fractures and a right temporal bone fracture with subarachnoid hemorrhage. Cerebellar and frontal lobe contusions were evident with diffuse axonal injury. An electroencephalogram was normal with no epileptiform activity.

Progress

Six years following the TBI, she was maintained on a monthly haloperidol depot injection with partial response. She did not believe the depot was helping and felt bullied into taking this medication, which took her pride away. Previously, she had tried several other oral antipsychotics with early effect but eventually became non-concordant. She was finally switched to a depot to ensure compliance. In the time following the first appearance of delusional thoughts, she continued to express paranoid beliefs. For instance, she believed the eye surgery was part of a cover-up for the implanted microchip and that she was kidnapped and locked on a hospital ward. Her preoccupation with the cranially implanted electronic device, however, lessened on medication. Overall, her delusional symptoms were still of a degree to causing significant disability.

Diagnosis

In considering the differential diagnosis, one must exclude delirium, substance-induced psychosis, or post-traumatic stress disorder (PTSD) from the list of potential candidates. The former is by definition an acute and transient state and contrary to her presentation. She did abuse alcohol to a degree, but the timeline or history does not suggest the emergence of psychotic symptoms having developed during or after alcohol consumption and there are no medical records documenting withdrawal. Psychotic symptoms in PTSD are largely event related and have an earlier onset, and again, this was not seen in this presentation [1, 2]. Schizophrenia, generally regarded as a neurodevelopmental disorder, may be a more likely diagnosis; however, she had never experienced any psychotic symptoms pre-TBI, she is middle aged, and there is no family history of schizophrenia or other mental disorders [3]. Still, TBI may be a risk factor in individuals with a genetic predisposition to developing schizophrenia, but without the genetic vulnerability present, this association becomes increasingly less probable [4, 5]. The most likely diagnosis appears to be a psychotic disorder due to TBI, i.e., an organic delusional (schizophrenia-like) disorder. This is further supported by a mean latency in presentation of 4–5 years post-TBI, paranoid delusions, focal lesions in the frontal lobe, as well as cognitive deficits in relation to executive and memory function [6, 7].

What Did I Learn from This Case?

I learned that psychotic presentations post-TBI can have a latency of several years and that an organic post-TBI psychosis may be more resistant to antipsychotic treatment as opposed to a psychotic disorder due to a neurodevelopmental origin. The accompanying severe cognitive deficits further complicate the mental state, limiting hopes for a more positive recovery from the psychosis.

References

1. American Psychiatric Association, DSM-5 Task Force. Diagnostic and statistical manual of mental disorders: DSM-5. 5th ed. Washington, DC: American Psychiatric Association; 2013. xliv, 947 p. p.
2. World Health Organization. The ICD-10 classification of mental and behavioural disorders: clinical descriptions and diagnostic guidelines. Geneva: World Health Organization; 1992. xii, 362 p. p.
3. Rapoport JL, Giedd JN, Gogtay N. Neurodevelopmental model of schizophrenia: update 2012. Mol Psychiatry. 2012;17(12):1228–38.
4. Kim E. Does traumatic brain injury predispose individuals to develop schizophrenia? Curr Opin Psychiatry. 2008;21(3):286–9.
5. Harrison G, Whitley E, Rasmussen F, Lewis G, Dalman C, Gunnell D. Risk of schizophrenia and other non-affective psychosis among individuals exposed to head injury: case control study. Schizophr Res. 2006;88(1–3):119–26.
6. Fujii D, Fujii DC. Psychotic disorder due to traumatic brain injury: analysis of case studies in the literature. J Neuropsychiatry Clin Neurosci. 2012;24(3):278–89.
7. Sachdev P, Smith JS, Cathcart S. Schizophrenia-like psychosis following traumatic brain injury: a chart-based descriptive and case-control study. Psychol Med. 2001;31(2):231–9.

Chapter 38
Bilateral Lesions of the Thalamus: A Neuropsychiatric Challenge

Lars Wojtecki and Alfons Schnitzler

Initial Investigations and Treatment

We report on a 75-year-old male retired school teacher who developed subacute deficits in orientation over the course of 2 weeks. Due to MRI findings that indicated hemorrhagic transformation and edema of both thalami together with a slight CSF pleocytosis, the patient was treated by the referring hospital with acyclovir against viral encephalitis.

Clinical Examination

On admission to our hospital, the patient was disorientated concerning place, time, person, and situation. He was friendly in personal contact and showed adequate affect. He showed a strong tendency to confabulation and perseveration alongside with anosognosia. He had no clinical signs of meningism and no headache. Hand coordination showed dysdiadochokinesia. Walking showed slight ataxia. There was intention tremor and action tremor of both hands.

L. Wojtecki, MD • A. Schnitzler, MD (✉)
Department of Neurology, Institute of Clinical Neuroscience and Medical Psychology, Universitätsklinikum Düsseldorf, Düsseldorf, Germany
e-mail: wojtecki@uni-duesseldorf.de; schnitza@uni-duesseldorf.de

J. Priller, H. Rickards (eds.), *Neuropsychiatry Case Studies*,
DOI 10.1007/978-3-319-42190-2_38

Neuropsychological examination showed short- and long-term memory deficits especially in the verbal domain. Furthermore, executive functions and visuoconstructive abilities were strongly affected.

Imaging

Cranial MRI showed T2*-hypointense signals in both medial thalami with a stronger affection of the left hemisphere. T2- and FLAIR-weighted MRI showed hyperintense thalamic signals. There was no gadolinium contrast enhancement in the T1 sequences. Taken together, the MRI was suspicious of a hemorrhagic transformation and edema of the thalami. MRI, CT (both including angiography), and ultrasound gave no evidence of vascular abnormalities of the arteries and veins.

Differential Diagnosis and Further Examinations

A second workup of the CSF revealed an unspecific slight pleocytosis and protein increase with negative results for various infections including Borrelia, Treponema, toxoplasmosis, CMV, HHV, HSV, VZV, EBV, FSME, Rickettsia, Brucella and Japanese encephalitis, and West Nile virus (the patient had been traveling weeks before disease onset). Thus, the hypothesis of virus encephalitis was withdrawn.

Although imaging of the edema was regredient under steroid treatment, there was no evidence for an autoimmune encephalitis with negative vasculitis screening, normal IgG Index, and no oligoclonal bands. Antineuronal antibodies were also negative, and vitamin levels were normal. A detailed tumor screening was negative. Flow cytometry of the CSF showed no abnormal cells.

After careful reconsideration of the MRI findings (for review, see [1]) and despite the absence of direct imaging evidence, we started anticoagulation with heparin under the diagnosis of a thrombosis of the deep thalamic veins. D-dimeres and thrombophilia screening was negative.

Disease Course

Despite anticoagulation treatment, the patient deteriorated in his condition. He showed altered states of vigilance with two episodes of sopor after sudden verbal aggressions. Mood state changed to a persistent anhedonia and depressive condition. EEG examination showed a slowed basic rhythm and bifrontal sharp waves. We diagnosed complex focal seizures and started treatment with lacosamide bridged with lorazepam. At this stage, MRI showed new signs of thalamic blood-brain barrier alterations after application of gadolinium. Furthermore, there was increased perifocal edema leading to a compression of the ventricle and consecutive hydrocephalus. Three differential diagnoses besides venous thrombosis with secondary hemorrhagic transformation and venous infarction were reconsidered: (1) infection, (2) tumor (lymphoma), and (3) a distinct entity called subacute diencephalic angioencephalopathy (SDAE) [2]. Thus, stereotactic biopsy was done. The neuropathological workup showed edema, astrogliosis, activated microglia, microangiopathy (also with thickening of vessel walls), no neoplasia, and no infection. The findings were not considered typical for SDAE due to missing necrosis of the parenchyma.

Diagnosis

As shown above, after careful workup most differential diagnoses were ruled out. Thus, the treatment of a venous thrombosis was maintained. In the postoperative follow-up, another MRI with MR angiography was done, which now proved the thrombosis in the sinus rectus and vein of Rosenthal on the left side. Over the course of months, imaging showed a slow improvement of the thalamic lesions (Fig. 38.1).

What Did We Learn from This Case?

First, we find the case very instructive concerning the many possible clinical presentations of thalamic affections. Besides causing hyperkinetic movements (here action and intention tremor), affection of the thalamus can lead to various neuropsychiatric manifestations. The thalamus – especially the here-affected medial part – is crucial for cognitive functions, including memory processing, attention, and orientation [3]. All these functions were altered in the abovementioned patient. Furthermore, vigilance and affect were altered and complex partial seizures were diagnosed. Second, the case is very instructive for the various neuroradiological differential diagnoses of thalamic lesions [1]. Especially challenging was the proof of a venous thrombosis of smaller vessels which can be sometimes limited due to technical constraints. The fact that the edema responded partly to steroid treatment led us to reconsider the possibility of a lymphoma, which could not be found in CSF or biopsy. However, cerebral biopsy in unclear cases without prompt response to treatment should always be considered.

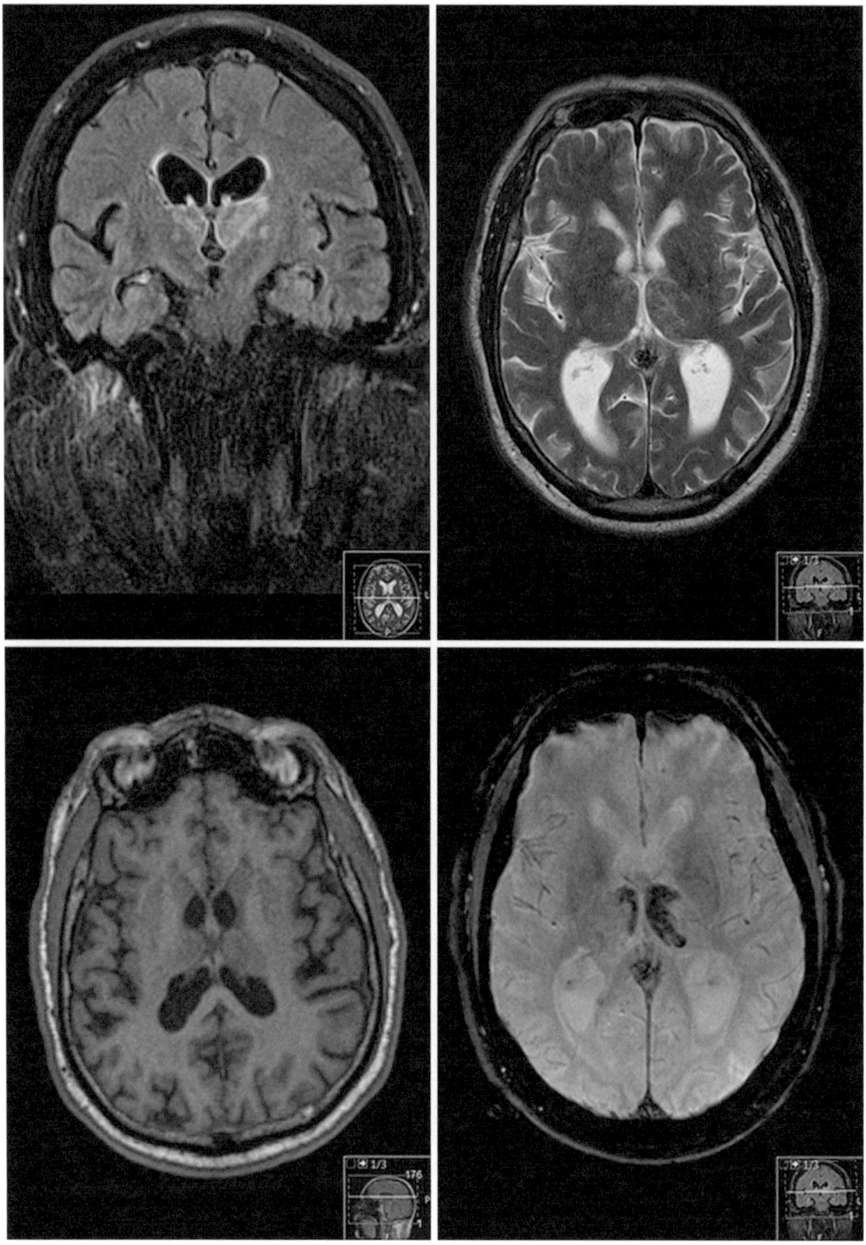

Fig. 38.1 MRI of the bithamalic lesions. *Top row left*: coronary FLAIR, hyperintense signal predominantly in the left thalamus. *Top row right*: axial T2-hyperintense signal. *Bottom row left*: axial T1-iso-/hypointense signal. *Bottom row right*: T2*-hypointense signal

References

1. Hegde AN, Mohan S, Lath N, Lim CCT. Differential diagnosis for bilateral abnormalities of the basal ganglia and thalamus. Radiographics. 2011;31:5–30.
2. Tihan T, Burger PC, Pomper M, Sanchez O, Ramzan M, Eberhart CG, et al. Subacute diencephalic angioencephalopathy: biopsy diagnosis and radiological features of a rare entity. Clin Neurol Neurosurg. 2001;103:160–7.
3. Saalmann YB. Intralaminar and medial thalamic influence on cortical synchrony, information transmission and cognition. Front Syst Neurosci. 2014;8:83.

Chapter 39
Listening to the Music and the Patient

Jan Adriaan Coebergh

Background History

The 52-year-old patient has had reduced hearing since 1993. She is currently fully deaf on the right, and the left is significantly impaired. She has had hearing aids since 10 years. She briefly took an SSRI a few years ago when she had episodes of low mood.

Since 2 or 3 years, one day, she has started hearing music. There have been hundreds of songs from the time when she was hearing like Queen, Fleetwood Mac, and Beatles, and the only modern one is Michael Bublé which is in her range of hearing. She can hear the same song for three consecutive mornings. It is present from the moment she wakes up and stops just after finishing a sentence. It used to be only present when quiet and now is distressing because it is stressful to keep trying to avoid being distracted by it. The songs are only parts of a song that then will repeat endlessly until she tries to change it. For many years, she did not tell anyone because she thought people would think she was crazy, and she only told her partner (who she has known 2 years) 6 months ago. She has no tinnitus. She has never sung along. It does interfere with falling asleep, but if she reads the same page three times, it can turn the music off. Watching television does improve it, but adjusting hearing aids has not made a difference. There are no other sounds or voices. It is at the level of conversation in volume. It is experienced in external space, and there are no other hallucinations. She was musical; she used to be singing in a choir and playing the guitar and violin.

J.A. Coebergh, MBBS, FRCP
Department of Neurology, Ashford St Peter's Foundation NHS Trust, Chertsey, UK
e-mail: jcoebergh@hotmail.com

J. Priller, H. Rickards (eds.), *Neuropsychiatry Case Studies*,
DOI 10.1007/978-3-319-42190-2_39

Her sleep has been horrible where she wakes up because of hot flushes (in the menopause), and then she has to fight the music. She has a fear that the music will catch up on her, and one day she will wake up and cannot cope. There are some current stressors like shoulder operations and illness in her elderly mother.

She is on indomethacin 25 mg bd and omeprazole since 6 months and is on the pill.

She works as a care home manager, and there are no significant intoxications.

Examination

Her neurological examination and mental state examination were normal. She started hearing music after a few seconds after stopping conversation which was an old Western "Crazy For You" that apparently she used to listen to.

Initial Investigations

Routine MRI head and laboratory investigations were normal.

Progress

I explained the nature of musical hallucinations and assuaged fears of mental illness. We discussed the effect of mood and sleep and further explored environmental measures (that she had discovered already but were insufficiently helpful). I recommended *Musicophilia* by Oliver Sacks as further reading. We then discussed pharmacological treatment. Based on my experience with approximately 30 patients and review of 147 articles discussing treatment in 276 individuals, I suggest acetylcholinesterase inhibitors. They have the highest published response rate and are generally tolerated well.

Since starting the rivastigmine first at 1.5 mg once a day, and then at BD, she had four to five periods where it was quite for up to 20 min which gave her an elated feeling. This occurred when she was calm, happy, and relaxed. There has been no change in volume, but there has been a change in music of previously clearly hearing proper lyrics where now she is just hearing a brief melody. She finds it more difficult to change the tunes. It has not changed her spontaneous residual inhibition of 1 s of starting after sounds like talking stop.

On increasing the dose, the patient wrote: "Since I have been taking 6 mg/day (3mg BD) of the Rivastigmine there is virtually no change in the hallucinations, their frequency of intensity. If anything, they are more intense in that the repetition of lyrics or music is shorter. For example, I may have one line or a short segment of a melody repeating itself until I am either distracted by conversation or I work hard at changing to another song. The "quiet moments" as I call them have been very sporadic and random. The only change is that on the few occasions I have had them, they do last longer, the longest having been approximately two hours. I have tried to see that as a positive, but in the past ten days, I have had only two or three quiet moments. I question whether staying on the Rivastigmine is beneficial."

Diagnosis

Musical hallucinations in the presence of hearing loss.

Further Considerations

A recent review of treatment that demonstrates a large amount of pharmacological interventions has been published, and in the idiopathic group, a next step would be antiepileptics (she is now starting carbamazepine). Environmental interventions like a tinnitus mask and psychological interventions like CBT have rarely been used but should be explored further. Cochlear implantation has been known to cause musical hallucinations, so she is reluctant to explore it further now. If completely treatment resistant and troublesome, rTMS should be explored, after publication of one case report.

The literature on treatment of musical hallucinations frequently does not discuss in detail what improvements are and how meaningful they are to the patient. In this case, a loss of control and occasionally quiet moments is a change, but not a meaningful one. The literature on treatment of musical hallucinations in all likelihood suffers from a positive publication bias, both of patients desiring/given treatment and of good treatment responses. No prospective large series are available to inform natural history and desire for and response to treatment.

Musical hallucinations are unusual hallucinations in that they are frequently and are so clearly suppressed by external input, and sometimes patients have the ability to switch songs. The pathophysiology is diverse, but a recent article describing altered multiple network processing seems to be consistent with the diverse phenomenology.

What Did I Learn from This Case?

Musical hallucinations can be a significant burden, and the phenomenology, natural history, and desire for and meaningful response to treatment remain enigmatic. Listening to the patient is essential to devise individualized treatment plans.

Bibliography

Blom JD, Coebergh JA, Lauw R, Sommer IE. Musical hallucinations treated with acetylcholinesterase inhibitors. Front Psychiatry. 2015;6:46.

Coebergh JA, Lauw R, Bots, R, Sommer IE, Blom JD. Musical hallucinations: review of treatment effects. Front Psychol. 2015 (Submitted for publication).

Cosentino G, Giglia G, Palermo A, Panetta ML, Lo Baido R, Brighina F, Fierro B. A case of post-traumatic complex auditory hallucinosis treated with rTMS. Neurocase. 2010;16(3):267–72.

Kumar S, Sedley W, Barnes GR, Teki S, Friston KJ, Griffiths TD. A brain basis for musical hallucinations. Cortex. 2014;52:86–97.

Chapter 40
Autistic Disorder in Neurofibromatosis

Stefanie C. Linden

D, who is 25 years old, had been diagnosed with neurofibromatosis type I (NF1) at the age of 4. He inherited the disease from his mother who is only mildly affected. D has a plexiform neuroma of the sciatic nerve and neuromas affecting his optic nerves. He has suffered from constant pain and coordination and balance problems since his early years. D was referred to a specialist service for adult autism because his parents suspected Asperger's syndrome.

Background History

D was born 5.5 weeks premature and weighed 4.7 lbs. His motor and language development were delayed, and he received speech therapy. He could only close his buttons at the age of 10–11 and tie his shoe laces in his teens. His balance was always impaired, and he could never run. D always struggled with writing and counting – he could not write his own name at the age of 6. D initially attended a mainstream school, and from the age of 6, he was referred to a Special Needs Unit. He had concentration problems but did not struggle particularly with academic material. He only had one very close friend who was considerably younger than him. His father recounts that D always looked out for younger children. At the age of 13, he required a spinal fusion operation for scoliosis. The long periods in hospital were disruptive to his schooling, and he left school without formal

S.C. Linden, MD, PhD
Institute of Psychological Medicine and Clinical Neurosciences,
Cardiff University School of Medicine, Cardiff, UK
e-mail: LindenS@cardiff.ac.uk

J. Priller, H. Rickards (eds.), *Neuropsychiatry Case Studies*,
DOI 10.1007/978-3-319-42190-2_40

qualifications. However, he obtained a national diploma at college and graduated from a foundation course in art, media, and design. D works as an extra in television productions and takes part in drama projects. He is also a blogger and has his own show on the local radio.

Examination

D engaged well in the conversation and described his mood as "good." He showed normal emotional reactivity and modulation. D reported that he can be irritable and sometimes had a vage feeling of people plotting against him, but there was no evidence of psychotic symptoms. D reported some compulsive behaviors, for example, checking switches and windows. There was no evidence of specific phobias, agoraphobia, or generalized anxiety, but he gets quite distressed when in big crowds and is overwhelmed in complex social situations.

Interview with Informant (Mother)

D has difficulties developing, maintaining, and understanding relationships. As a child, D only interacted with considerably younger children. He now interacts more with his own age group. Most of his friends have a diagnosis of autism spectrum disorder. D does not pick up on sarcasm or irony and sometimes "does not get the subtle cues" in a conversation. However, in his adult years, D has learned to make eye contact with his friends. He is very sensitive to sounds and temperature.

D does not use emotionally expressive gestures; he would not hug or put his arm around another person to show sympathy. He does not have a wide range of facial expressions and hardly ever smiles. He uses little body language and expressive gestures and generally tries to avoid body contact. He does not like to be comforted by others even for his frequent bouts of pain. He has learned to identify when other people are distressed, but he generally does not understand why they are upset. He frequently does not understand what other people try to tell him. This misunderstanding of other people's motives has caused considerable tension in social situations.

When younger, D had a fascination for small objects; he always had to hold something in his hand, and he liked to turn these objects around in his hand. He is now a keen collector of memorabilia of science fiction television programs and movies. D gets extremely upset when somebody else changes his plans or routines. When he was a child, he was obsessed with certain foods. He would only eat one particular dish for a certain period time. Until today, different foods have to be strictly separated on his plate.

Conclusion

D has deficits in social-emotional reciprocity and nonverbal communicative behaviors and a restricted pattern of behavior and interests, which started in his early developmental period. He thus meets the DSM-5 criteria for a mild form of autism spectrum disorder (ASD), which is also commonly described as Asperger's syndrome. A central question both for the clinical team and the patient and his family was whether this psychiatric phenotype was related to any detectable brain pathology arising from the NF1 disease process.

Investigations

The family informed us that a routine MRI of the head, conducted at a national reference center for NF1, did not show any abnormalities in the brain.

What Did I Learn from This Case?

ASD is relatively common in NF1. Reported prevalence rates of ASD in NF1 are in the range of approximately 20–40 % [1–3], which is considerably higher than the estimated population prevalence of ASD (1 %). Features of autism seem to be equally prominent in NF1 patients with and without brain tumors [4] although this evidence is still preliminary because of small patient numbers, and further investigations into the pathophysiology of ASD in NF1 and specific genotype-phenotype correlations are needed. For clinicians it is important to be aware of the likely underreporting and underdiagnosis of ASD and other psychiatric phenotypes in NF1 and other genetic syndromes [1].

References

1. Garg S, Green J, Leadbitter K, et al. Neurofibromatosis type 1 and autism spectrum disorder. Pediatrics. 2013;132(6):e1642–8.
2. Richards C, Jones C, Groves L, Moss J, Oliver C. Prevalence of autism spectrum disorder phenomenology in genetic disorders: a systematic review and meta-analysis. Lancet Psychiatry. 2015;2(10):909–16.
3. Garg S, Plasschaert E, Descheemaeker MJ, et al. Autism spectrum disorder profile in neurofibromatosis type I. J Autism Dev Disord. 2015;45(6):1649–57.
4. Constantino JN, Zhang Y, Holzhauer K, et al. Distribution and within-family specificity of quantitative autistic traits in patients with neurofibromatosis type I. J Pediatr. 2015;167(3):621–626.e621.

Chapter 41
Case Vignette: When You Can't Make Sense of the Story

Hilary Lloyd

T was referred for a psychiatric assessment from the pediatric ward at the age of 12 years. He had been admitted from the emergency department because of a 2–3-day history of being quieter than usual, appearing to be "in a different world" and not making complete sense in conversation. He had presented to his GP a week previously with symptoms of an upper respiratory tract infection, with cough, for which he had been prescribed amoxicillin. T said that he felt "like I did before." On examination, he appeared to be somewhat agitated and perplexed, but no clear psychotic features were evident. He appeared to have fully recovered within 4 days (the whole episode having lasted 6 days) and was discharged home.

Within 3 weeks, T presented in a similar state, again to pediatrics through the emergency department. He was readmitted. He had complained that he could not see properly, was tired, and appeared to be exhausted. His conversation was vague, and he often said he could not remember when he was asked questions. On the ward, he slept and rested, waking to eat. His affect appeared to be "odd," and his behavior was often "abrupt" with unpredictable shouting and repeating of questions.

Background History

T had been a normally developing pubescent boy. He was well socialized and popular and academically able, attending a local independent (competitive entry) high school. He enjoyed football. He was the older of a sibship of 2. He was born in the Netherlands, his parents having been refugees from the conflict in a central African country. T had never visited the African continent.

H. Lloyd, MB, ChB, FRCPsych
Child & Adolescent Mental Health Services, Royal Manchester Children's Hospital, Manchester, UK
e-mail: hilary.lloyd@cmft.nhs.uk

J. Priller, H. Rickards (eds.), *Neuropsychiatry Case Studies*,
DOI 10.1007/978-3-319-42190-2_41

There was no previous psychiatric history. T had experienced a single, brief (5 days) similar episode 2 years previously, following an upper respiratory tract infection and the prescription of amoxicillin. He was admitted to a pediatric ward at this time. The episode resolved spontaneously, and the diagnosis was of idiopathic confusional state.

Medical investigations included urea and electrolytes, thyroid function, full blood count, liver function, serum copper, autoantibodies (including anti-NMDA), metabolic screen, MR head, and standard EEG. All were normal.

Examination

When seen by the psychiatrist, he was rousable but tired and spoke in short sentences. There was no evidence of formal thought disorder, and he was fully orientated but appeared rather "obtunded." There were no systematized delusions, but T expressed some anxiety at the prospect of his father leaving the ward and gave "Something might happen to us and we might die" as the reason for this. He said, "We might die of confusion" when asked how he and his mother might die if his father left the ward. He said to the psychiatrist, "You are frightening me. I haven't seen you before."

Initial Differential Diagnosis

The general pediatrician was of the view that T's presentation was entirely within the "mental health" domain. T was transferred to the children's psychiatric unit. He continued to appear rather drowsy but rousable on the unit. He complained that his vision was "not quite right." He remained fully orientated and cooperative. His parents were concerned about his tiredness. An ophthalmology assessment revealed no abnormal findings. T recovered to his previous level of functioning within a total of 15 days from its onset. He remained on the mental health unit for a further 2 weeks (with home leave) and, having remained well, was discharged home and to his local CAMHS for follow-up. This episode lasted 15 days in total. The pediatrician did not offer follow-up. The differential diagnosis considered at this point was psychotic episodes ("boufee delirante"), dissociative disorder, and acute confusional state of unknown etiology. T's parents remained cooperative but concerned that there was an underlying, missed medical explanation for T's symptoms.

Progress

T had a further episode 4 months later, lasting 20 days, and one more after a further 2 months, lasting 10 days. During each episode, he did not attend school because of difficulties in concentrating. He appeared tired and lassitudinous.

A further episode occurred after another 2 months, and the psychiatrist saw him frequently during this period. No reinforcers or gains of the episodes were evident. The episodes involved weekends as well as school days and occurred during holidays. They did not involve the school examination period. There was no delusional ideation during the episodes, and there was no affective symptomatology. During visits to the clinic, T remained awake but slouched in his chair, appeared apathetic, and contributed to the conversation only when pressed, a marked difference from his normal self. He was slow to answer questions, and, at times, his thoughts were difficult to follow, although his orientation remained intact. There was no evidence of hallucinations. The episodes were not understandable in psychodynamic terms. In between the discrete episodes, he returned to his normal, high-functioning state. The pattern was not typical of a developing serious mental illness.

Reassessment and Joint Working

The psychiatrist therefore discussed the case with a pediatric neurology colleague, requesting a second opinion, and a joint appointment was arranged. The neurologist reviewed the medical investigations already done and suggested a porphyrin screen and prolonged EEG during the next episode. Arrangements were agreed for T to be admitted under the neurology team during the next episode so that he could be observed and the investigations completed, and the psychiatrist would do regular mental state examinations.

Diagnosis

The porphyrin screen was normal, and the EEG showed only excessive sleep, as did the direct observations. Mental state findings were similar to those in the previous episode. When T had recovered from the episode, he described having felt as though he had been dreaming and appeared to be describing experiences of derealization. The pediatric neurologist suggested a diagnosis of Kleine-Levin syndrome. Overeating had not been a prominent feature of the episodes, but T had been hungry when he recovered and had a tendency to uncharacteristically request carbohydrate-heavy foods. There was no hypersexuality.

T was now aged 13 years. On review of the evidence, and somewhat wary of commencing lithium therapy in a child of this age, the pediatric neurologist and psychiatrist advised a therapeutic trial of carbamazepine. This was commenced some 12 months after T's first presentation to the pediatric ward. Over the following 15 months, he had a further six episodes, lasting between 4 and 10 days (see Fig. 41.1). His parents reported that these episodes appeared to be less severe than the previous ones.

T's parents then took the opportunity to consult with a world expert in Kleine-Levin syndrome, who recommended a therapeutic trial of lithium. This was instituted by the psychiatrist, following the protocol advised. The aim is to

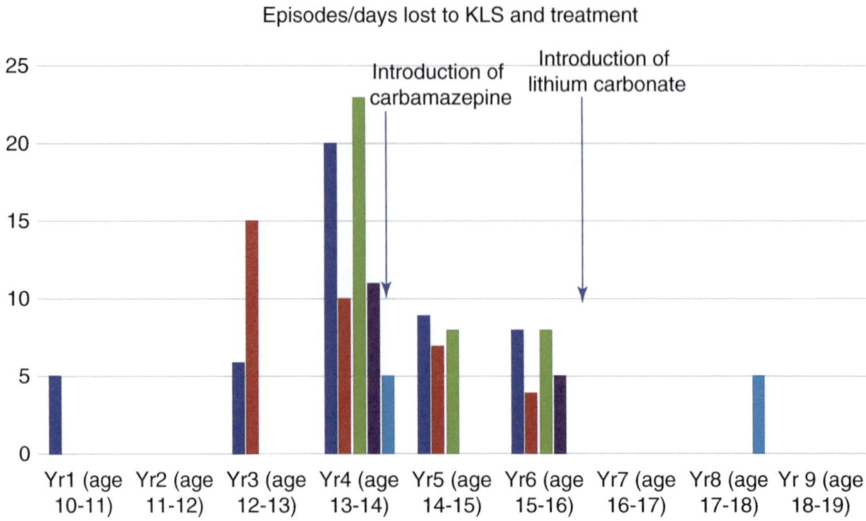

Fig. 41.1 Episodes/days lost to KLS. Year 1: one episode of 5 days – total 5 days. Year 2: no episodes – total 0 days. Year 3: two episodes (6 and 15 days) – total 21 days. Year 4: five episodes (20, 10, 23, 11, and 5 days) – carbamazepine introduced between fourth and fifth episodes – total 69 days. Year 5: three episodes (9, 7, and 8 days) – total 24 days. Year 6: four episodes (8, 4, 8, and 5 days) – lithium introduced after fourth episode – total 25 days. Year 7: no episodes – total 0 days. Year 8: one episode (5 days) – total 5 days. Year 9: no episodes – total 0 days

continue the lithium therapy until 3 years after the last episode. Since the introduction of the lithium, there has been a marked reduction in episodes; only one has occurred 2 years after its introduction (see Fig. 41.1). In the interim, T was able to successfully study for and sit his GCSE and A-level examinations and has progressed onto a degree course.

What Did I Learn from This Case?

When symptoms and course do not make sense, step back and reassess. Do not be afraid to challenge a physician's view that something is entirely within the "mental health realm" – seek an appropriate second opinion/consult a colleague if necessary.

Kleine-Levin is a rare and poorly understood syndrome, often affecting adolescent males [1]. The diagnostic criteria used in the International Classification of Sleep Disorders (revision 2, 2005) are given in Table 41.1. Although the syndrome itself may be seen as being benign and tends to resolve spontaneously after a mean duration of 14 years, the episodes can be highly disruptive to study and academic achievement at a crucial stage of life. Therefore, lithium therapy is worth considering (which has the strongest evidence base in KLS) [1–3].

Table 41.1 Diagnostic criteria of Kleine-Levin syndrome

International classification of sleep disorders – revision 2 (2005)
Recurrent hypersomnia
Recurrent episodes of excessive daytime sleepiness lasting 2 days to 4 weeks
Episodes recur at least once per year
Alertness, cognitive function, and behavior are normal between episodes
Hypersomnia is not explained by another sleep, medical, neurological or psychiatric disorder, medication use, or substance abuse
In addition to the recurrent hypersomnia criteria, the patient should have at least one of the following
Cognitive abnormalities, e.g., confusion, derealization, hallucinations
Abnormal behavior – irritability, aggression
Hyperphagia
Hypersexuality

In this case, while the diagnosis of KLS was made by a pediatric neurology colleague, the psychiatrist is best placed to treat because of familiarity with lithium therapy.

KLS has many mental state manifestations, and the exclusion of serious mental illness may be an important role of the psychiatrist [4].

Joint working between psychiatrist and physicians, with avoidance of the "over to you" split, remains highly valuable and rewarding to patients.

Bibliography

1. Arnulf I, Zeitzer JM, File J, Farber N, Mignol E. Kleine-Levin syndrome: a systematic review of 186 cases in the literature. Brain. 2005;128(Pt 12):2763–76.
2. Arnulf I, Rico TJ, Mignot E. Diagnosis, disease course, and management of patients with Kleine-Levin syndrome. Lancet Neurol. 2012;11(10):918–28.
3. Leur-Semenescu S, Le Corvec T, Groos E, Lavault S, Golmard JL, Arnulf I. Lithium therapy in Kleine-Levin syndrome: an open-label, controlled study in 130 patients. Neurology. 2015; 85(19):1655–62.
4. Millichap JG. Differential diagnosis of Kleine-Levin syndrome. Paediatr Neurol. 2015;29(3):24.

MIX
Papier aus verantwortungsvollen Quellen
Paper from responsible sources
FSC® C105338

If you have any concerns about our products,
you can contact us on
ProductSafety@springernature.com

In case Publisher is established outside the EU,
the EU authorized representative is:
Springer Nature Customer Service Center GmbH
Europaplatz 3, 69115 Heidelberg, Germany

Printed by Libri Plureos GmbH
in Hamburg, Germany